52 FOODS AND SUPPLEMENTS

FOR A HEALTHY HEART

52 FOODS AND SUPPLEMENTS

FOR A HEALTHY HEART

Deborah Mitchell

A Lynn Sonberg Book

St. Martin's Paperbacks

Notice: This book is intended as a reference volume only, not as a medical manual. The information given here is designed to help you make informed decisions about your health. It is not intended as a substitute for any treatment that may have been prescribed by your doctor. If you suspect that you have a medical problem, we urge you to seek competent medical help.

Mention of specific companies, organizations, or authorities in this book does not imply endorsement by the author or publisher, nor does mention of specific companies, organizations, or authorities imply that they endorse this book, its author or the publisher.

Internet addresses given in this book were accurate at the time it went to press.

52 FOODS AND SUPPLEMENTS FOR A HEALTHY HEART

Copyright © 2010 by Lynn Sonberg Book Associates.

Cover photo by Getty Images / Lew Robertson.

All rights reserved.

For information address St. Martin's Press, 175 Fifth Avenue, New York, NY 10010.

EAN: 978-0-312-37315-3

Printed in the United States of America

St. Martin's Paperbacks edition / February 2010

St. Martin's Paperbacks are published by St. Martin's Press, 175 Fifth Avenue, New York, NY 10010.

10 9 8 7 6 5 4 3 2 1

CONTENTS

INTRODUCTION

You have the power to prevent heart disease, and you can do it easily, every day, three times a day. Yes, you can eat to save your heart.

In April 2009, a comprehensive study appeared in the *Archives of Internal Medicine*. The authors had conducted a systematic search and evaluation of studies and trials that had investigated the association between diet and coronary heart disease between 1950 and 2007. The undertaking involved the analysis of nearly 200 studies involving millions of people, and the results were clear and strong: If you want a healthy heart, you should follow the Mediterranean diet pattern, which is rich in fruits, vegetables, nuts, legumes, whole grains, cereals, olive oil, fish, and wine (in moderation on the wine!), and low in meat, dairy foods, junk food, and fat.

This way of eating includes lots of vitamins, minerals, and phytonutrients (plant nutrients). The study also noted that it was best to get essential nutrients such as vitamins C and E, beta-carotene, folic acid, and fiber from your food and not from supplements. On the "no-no" food list were starchy carbohydrates like white bread and foods that contain trans fat, which is present in fried fast foods and many cookies, crackers, processed and frozen foods, and snack foods.

This book is an extension of that study, and more. It is a handy, comprehensive, and delicious (yes, we have recipes) way to eat for a healthy heart. Along the way we provide information on heart disease today, its risk factors, how to prevent heart disease, and how it is treated. But the main message is how to eat to keep your heart healthy.

HOW TO USE THIS BOOK

We suggest that you read through the first three chapters so you can get a clearer understanding of heart disease and the impact it can have on your life and the lives of your loved ones. These chapters provide essential information that can help make you better prepared to talk to your doctor about heart disease.

Chapter 4 introduces 40 heart-healthy foods, and you can use the chapter in two ways. You can look up foods that you already enjoy and learn about their heart-healthy properties. But we also hope you will explore some new foods and add them to your diet. After all, we give you easy, delicious recipes to entice you!

Chapter 5 is helpful if you are considering adding heart-healthy supplements to your life. We encourage you to take this book with you when you visit your doctor so you can discuss these supplements.

Chapter 6 is self-explanatory: seven days of menu ideas that include the recipes offered in chapter 4. At the end of the book, note that there are references for the scientific research that supports the use of both the foods and supplements discussed in the book.

Enjoy!

PART I

Welcome to Your Heart

CHAPTER 1

Everyone Needs This Book:
Heart Disease Today

Chances are you or someone you love is at risk for heart disease right now. No, we don't say this to scare you, although we do want to get your attention. Perhaps facts like these will cause you to pause: More than 785,000 Americans will experience a new coronary attack in 2009, and about 470,000 will have a repeat attack. Heart disease is the number one killer in the United States, and it is becoming an increasing problem among younger people.

Perhaps you have already heard some of this information, and maybe that's why you've picked up this book. We're glad you did, because we hope you are ready to take steps to prevent heart disease or, if it is already a presence in your life, incorporate measures to manage it in a healthy, tasty, and enjoyable way, every day of your life.

Before we get into the "how" of taking care of your heart, we begin with a discussion of the nuts and bolts of this vital organ and how it operates—and unfortunately doesn't operate for many people. So let's turn to your heart.

THE HEART OF THE MATTER

The human heart beats approximately 100,000 times each day, 365 days a year. Nearly 2,000 gallons of blood are transported through the heart each day, passing through nearly 100,000 miles of blood vessels. That's an incredible amount of work for one organ to do. For millions of people, the heart has some difficulty performing that work. That difficulty can manifest as different types of heart disease and its complications.

TYPES OF HEART DISEASE AND COMPLICATIONS

Heart disease is a general term used to describe a range of disorders that affect the heart and, in some cases, the blood vessels. Many people use the term "heart disease" interchangeably with "cardiovascular disease," a phrase that usually refers to conditions involving narrowed or blocked blood vessels that can cause a heart attack, stroke, or angina (chest pain).

Types of Heart Disease

Heart disease can refer to damage that occurs to many different structures, including the heart's valves, muscle, arteries, lining, and electrical circuitry. You can be born with a heart condition (inherited or congenital) or develop one—or more—later in life due to risk factors that you can control (e.g., diet, smoking, amount of exercise) or ones you cannot (age, ethnicity, gender). In addition, risk factors also can have an impact on inherited or congenital heart problems.

There are many different types of heart disease, and we give a brief explanation of the more common ones below.

- **Aneurysms.** When an artery is damaged and loses its elasticity and strength, it can develop a bulge called an aneurysm. The force of blood pushing against the weakened wall can cause the aneurysm to rupture, causing bleeding into and along the artery wall. A ruptured aneurysm is often fatal.

- **Angina.** This condition is marked by a feeling of pressure in the chest, shortness of breath, and sometimes sweating. Angina is a symptom of myocardial ischemia usually caused by coronary atherosclerosis (hardening of the arteries; *see below*).

- **Arrhythmia.** Any abnormal or disturbed heart rhythm is referred to as arrhythmia. This can include abnormally rapid (tachycardia), slow (bradycardia), or irregular rhythms.

- **Atherosclerosis.** This condition is commonly referred to as "hardening of the arteries" and is caused by an accumulation of cholesterol, fats, and other substances in the arteries. The buildup causes the arteries to become narrow and less flexible. Although loss of elasticity is a part of the aging process, factors such as smoking, diabetes, poor nutrition, and high blood pressure are also risk factors for atherosclerosis.

- **Cardiomyopathy.** Disease of the heart muscle. There are several types, including dilated cardiomyopathy and hypertrophic cardiomyopathy, which are explained below.

- **Congenital heart disease.** These conditions develop before birth. The most common types are obstruction of blood flow in the heart or vessels around the heart, an irregular pattern of blood flow through the heart, and various structural problems such as having just one ventricle instead of two. Approximately 36,000 infants are born with congenital heart disease each year.

- **Congestive heart failure.** If the heart is too damaged or weak to regulate blood flow properly, the blood can become congested in different locations (e.g., feet, lungs, legs) and cause swelling, as well as shortness of breath, paleness, and coolness in the legs and arms. These are symptoms of congestive heart failure.

- **Coronary artery disease.** This is the number one cause of heart attack. Coronary artery disease is a condition in which the heart muscle cannot get enough oxygen and blood. In addition to heart attack, coronary artery disease can lead to angina and, in severe cases, sudden death.

- **Diastolic dysfunction.** This is a type of heart failure in which the relaxation portion of the beat (diastolic) is abnormal. This abnormality prohibits the blood from flowing freely between the ventricles and sends it up into the arteries and veins. This action can cause swelling and increased pressure in the blood vessels of the lungs (pulmonary congestion) and/or in the blood vessels that enter the heart (systemic congestion).

• **Dilated cardiomyopathy.** If you have dilated cardiomyopathy, your heart muscles have become so weak and your heart chambers are so dilated that too much blood is released with every beat. This condition can be caused by coronary artery disease, myocarditis, or excessive alcohol use, or the reasons can be unknown.

• **Endocarditis.** A disease of the heart valves, endocarditis occurs when the endocardium (the membrane that lines the inside of the heart valves) becomes infected. Most cases develop as the result of surgery.

• **High blood pressure.** The force of blood on the artery walls as it is pumped through the body is blood pressure. If the flow is obstructed, the heart must pump more rapidly or with more force to push the blood through the vessels, causing blood pressure levels to rise. High blood pressure (hypertension) can lead to an aneurysm, an enlarged heart, or heart failure (*see above*).

• **Hypertrophic cardiomyopathy.** When the heart muscle becomes so thick that it restricts the amount of blood the ventricles can hold and pump, you have hypertrophic cardiomyopathy. This condition can result in sudden death and arrhythmia.

- **Mitral valve prolapse.** The mitral valve makes sure the blood flows toward the body during each beat. Mitral valve prolapse is an abnormality in which the valve goes backward as the heart contracts. The condition can progress gradually and the cause is unknown. In severe cases it can lead to congestive heart failure.

- **Myocardial ischemia.** Sometimes the blood supply to the myocardium (the muscular wall of the heart) is very low, which causes the heart muscle to function abnormally. An inadequate supply of blood is called ischemia. Because the heart muscle must work harder to try to get enough blood and oxygen, it can cause chest pain, shortness of breath, and fatigue. Angina is a symptom of myocardial ischemia.

- **Myocarditis.** An inflammation of the heart muscle (myocardium) is myocarditis. It is usually caused by a virus and characterized by fever, joint pain, chest pain, and an abnormally rapid heart rate.

- **Valve disease.** Any one or more of the four valves in the heart (mitral and aortic on the left side; tricuspid and pulmonary on the right) can become diseased. Diseased valves typically obstruct blood flow, become stiff and do not open easily, or fail to close properly, allowing blood to leak. A stiff (stenotic) valve reduces blood flow, causing the blood behind it to accumulate. This backup leads to symptoms of congestive heart failure and angina.

Valves that fail to close properly allow blood to leak back in the wrong direction, which may cause the heart chambers to enlarge. Weakened or damaged valves are susceptible to infections, called endocarditis (*see above*).

Complications of Heart Disease

The presence of heart disease is associated with a variety of complications. Here are the most common ones.

- **Heart attack.** Coronary artery disease can cause a heart attack. A heart attack, also referred to as a myocardial infarction, usually occurs when a blood clot blocks the flow of blood through a coronary artery. This interruption can damage or destroy a portion of the heart muscle.

- **Heart failure.** Heart failure occurs when the heart is unable to pump enough blood to meet the body's needs. What happens is this: As time goes on, the ventricles may become stiff and unable to fill with an adequate amount of blood between beats. The ventricles then stretch (dilate) so much that the heart can't pump blood efficiently throughout the body. The heart muscle also may become increasingly weak. Heart failure can result from many forms of heart disease, including cardiovascular disease, heart defects, valvular heart disease, and cardiomyopathy.

- **Peripheral artery disease.** This disease is typically caused by atherosclerosis. In cases of peripheral artery disease, the extremities—usually the legs—do not receive enough blood to keep up with demand. The most common symptom of peripheral artery disease is severe leg pain when walking. This is known as claudication, and since it often occurs intermittently, it is referred to as intermittent claudication.

- **Stroke.** A stroke, or cerebrovascular accident (CVA), occurs when the blood supply to the brain is interrupted, which stops the delivery of critical oxygen and glucose. Brain cells begin to die within just a few minutes of a stroke. A stroke most often is caused by a blood clot that travels to the arteries of the brain (ischemic stroke) or by bleeding (hemorrhage) in the brain from ruptured blood vessels.

- **Sudden cardiac arrest.** The sudden, unexpected loss of heart function, breathing, and consciousness is sudden cardiac arrest. This condition usually occurs when there is an electrical disturbance in the heart that interrupts its ability to pump blood, which abruptly stops blood flow to the body. Sudden cardiac arrest nearly always occurs as part of an underlying heart problem, especially coronary artery disease. Sudden cardiac arrest is fatal if not treated immediately.

WHO GETS HEART DISEASE?

Heart disease is an equal-opportunity condition: It can affect anyone at any age, from newborns to the very old. There was a time when most people assumed that heart disease occurred primarily in older adults, and to a great extent that is still true. However, because of the increasing prevalence of risk factors for heart disease among younger people, including obesity, type 2 diabetes, high cholesterol, and high blood pressure, we are seeing cases of heart disease develop in younger individuals.

Although heart disease is the number one killer of both men and women, and there are many similarities between the sexes when it comes to heart disease, there are also some important differences. We talk about some of those differences in chapter 2, for example, where we point out the signs and symptoms of heart disease, which can differ between men and women. Knowing those differences could save your life or that of a loved one someday.

Here we want to mention that women tend to experience heart disease ten years later than men, which is believed to be associated with the heart-protective effect of estrogen, and that they also tend to have a worse prognosis once they enter the hospital, which may be related to the fact that they tend to be older and/or have a more severe case by the time they are hospitalized. More women than men die of heart disease each year, and women are six times as likely to die of heart disease as of breast cancer. Heart disease kills more women older than 65 than do all types of cancer.

Heart Disease Statistics

According to the latest figures from the American Heart Association (the *2009 Heart Disease and Stroke Statistics,* which gives statistics for the latest years available, 2005–2006), these are the facts on the prevalence of heart disease and some of its risk factors and complications.

- **Coronary heart disease.** 16.8 million adults, or 7.6 percent of the adult population in the United

States. This includes 8.7 million men and 8.1 million women

- **Heart attack (myocardial infarction).** 7.9 million adults, including 4.7 million men and 3.2 million women

- **Heart failure.** 5.7 million adults, including 3.2 million men and 2.5 million women

- **High blood pressure.** 73.6 million adults, including 35.3 million men and 38.3 million women

- **High cholesterol** (200 mg/dL or higher). 98.6 million adults, including 45.0 million men and 53.6 million women

- **Obesity/overweight.** 145 million adults, including 76.9 million males and 68.1 million females

- **Stroke.** 6.5 million adults, including 2.6 million men and 3.9 million women

The website for this and more information is www.ameri canheart.org.

The risk of heart disease and its risk factors is not the same for each ethnic group. According to the HCHS NHSI 2007, the prevalence estimates for people age 18 and older are:

- Among whites, 11.4 percent have heart disease, 6.1 percent have coronary heart disease, 22.2

percent have hypertension, and 2.2 percent have had a stroke

- Among blacks or African Americans, 10.2 percent have heart disease, 6.0 percent have coronary heart disease, 31.7 percent have hypertension, and 3.7 percent have had a stroke

- Among Hispanics or Latinos, 8.8 percent have heart disease, 5.7 percent have coronary heart disease, 20.6 percent have hypertension, and 3.7 percent have had a stroke

- Among Asians, 6.9 percent have heart disease, 4.3 percent have coronary heart disease, 19.5 percent have hypertension, and 2.6 percent have had a stroke

Heart Disease in Children

Two types of heart disease are seen in children: congenital and acquired. Congenital heart disease, or congenital heart defect, is a condition that is present at birth. Each year, about 36,000 children in the United States are born with a heart defect. Examples include structural defects such as atrial septal defects, ventrical septal defects, and patent ductus arteriosis. Heart disease that develops during childhood (acquired heart disease) includes rheumatic fever, infective endocarditis, and Kawasaki disease.

High cholesterol in children is associated with three factors: heredity, obesity, and diet. Most children who have high cholesterol have a parent who also has hypercholesterolemia.

Higher than normal blood pressure is seen in about 20 percent of children, although less than 1 percent of children have significant hypertension (240 mg/dL or higher). In most cases, no cause can be identified. If hypertension becomes severe in children, it is usually a warning that there is a serious underlying problem, such as kidney disease, or abnormalities of the heart, endocrine (gland), or nervous system. If hypertension is not addressed or grows worse over the years, it can lead to heart failure or damage to the kidneys, eyes, and other organs.

RISK FACTORS FOR HEART DISEASE

When it comes to risk factors for heart disease, there are traditional factors that affect women and men about equally, and then there are those that tend to play a bigger role in the development of heart disease in women. We look at the risk factors for both sexes and note which ones tend to impact women more.

Overall in this section, however, we answer questions you, whether you are male or female, may have asked yourself about heart disease, namely:

- What are the chances that I will develop heart disease?

- What are the risk factors for heart disease?

- Are some risk factors more important than others?

- How many risk factors do I need to have before I should worry about getting heart disease?

Let's answer these important questions by looking at the types of risk factors for heart disease and how they can impact your health.

Major Risk Factors

Researchers have identified some factors as "major" because they significantly increase the risk of heart and blood vessel disease. Generally, the more risk factors you have, the greater your chance of developing coronary heart disease. In addition, the more severe level of each risk factor, the more that factor impacts your overall chances of getting cardiovascular disease.

Some major risk factors can't be changed. These include:

- **Increasing age.** Approximately 82 percent of people who die of coronary heart disease are 65 years or older. As people age, women who have a heart attack are more likely than men to die from them within a few weeks.

- **Gender.** Men are at greater risk of heart attacks than women, and they tend to have them at a younger age. Although women's rate of death from heart disease increases after menopause, it does not reach the level of men's.

- **Heredity and race.** If your parents had heart disease, you are more likely to develop it yourself. Because African Americans have more severe high blood pressure than whites, they also are at greater risk of heart disease. Other populations that have a higher risk of heart disease, in part due to their higher rates of obesity and diabetes, are Mexican Americans, Native Americans, native Hawaiians, and some Asian Americans.

It's important to remember that just because you can't change these risk factors, you can control others, and that can mean a great deal toward preventing heart disease. In the "Can Control" category (via lifestyle changes and/or treatment) are the following risk factors. We just mention them briefly here, because we discuss ways to prevent heart disease in more detail in chapter 3, "You Can Prevent Heart Disease."

• **Smoking.** People who smoke tobacco are at two to three times greater risk of dying from coronary heart disease than nonsmokers. Cigarette smoking also works synergistically with other risk factors to increase the risk for coronary heart disease. People who smoke pipes or cigars also have a significant risk of death from coronary heart disease, although it is somewhat less than among cigarette smokers. Smoking is a more significant risk factor for heart disease in women than in men.

• **High blood pressure.** Because high blood pressure makes the heart work harder, it increases the risk of heart attack, stroke, congestive heart failure, and kidney failure. If high blood pressure is present along with obesity, smoking, diabetes, and high cholesterol, the risk of having a heart attack or stroke increases several times.

- **Sedentary lifestyle.** Lack of regular physical activity is a risk factor for coronary heart disease. Physical activity helps control blood cholesterol, blood pressure, obesity, and diabetes—all risk factors for heart disease. Generally, the more vigorous the activity, the greater the benefits.

- **High blood cholesterol.** There is a direct relationship between a rise in blood cholesterol and risk of coronary heart disease. If you add other risk factors, the risk increases even more. Cholesterol level is affected by age, diet, family history, and gender.

- **Overweight/obesity.** The presence of excess body fat, especially if it is located around the waist, is a significant risk factor for heart disease and stroke, even if other risk factors are absent. The reason is that excess weight makes the heart work harder, which can raise blood pressure, cholesterol, and triglycerides. Being overweight also increases the chance that you will have diabetes.

- **Diabetes.** This disease significantly increases the risk of developing cardiovascular disease. The risk remains even if glucose levels are well managed, but the risks are even greater if blood sugar levels are not controlled. About 75 percent of people who have diabetes die of some type of cardiovascular disease.

- **Metabolic syndrome.** This syndrome is a combination of five metabolic risk factors for heart disease that tend to occur together. Metabolic syndrome is diagnosed when someone has at least three of these factors. They include excessive fat around the abdomen, high blood pressure, higher than normal blood sugar, higher than normal triglycerides, and lower than normal high-density lipoprotein cholesterol (HDL, the good cholesterol). Metabolic syndrome has a greater impact on women than on men.

- **High C-reactive protein levels.** This factor has not been officially placed in the "major" category as yet. C-reactive protein is a substance that indicates the presence of inflammation in the body. This is important because inflammation of the arteries has been linked to an increased risk of heart disease, heart attack, stroke, and peripheral arterial disease. A recent study (November 2008) found that high levels of C-reactive protein put patients at increased risk of developing cardiovascular disease. The findings of the study were so conclusive that the trial was stopped before its scheduled completion. The study's investigators believe the importance of C-reactive protein in increasing the risk of cardiovascular disease has been greatly underestimated, and that their findings stress the urgency of promoting this factor to "major" category.

Contributing Risk Factors

These risk factors contribute to but do not directly cause coronary heart disease.

- **Stress.** How you respond to stress may be a contributing factor. In fact, recent research is using neuroimaging techniques to illustrate and map the pathways that mechanistically link stressful experiences with the risk of coronary heart disease. Stress can also cause people to overeat, start smoking, or become too depressed to exercise. Mental stress and depression have a stronger impact on women's hearts than on men's. Depression is twice as common in women, and it increases the risk of heart disease by two to three times compared with women who are not depressed.

- **Alcohol use.** Excessive alcohol use can raise blood pressure and triglyceride levels, produce irregular heartbeats, and contribute to overweight. Moderate alcohol use, however, compared with no alcohol use, is associated with a reduced risk. Moderate use is defined as one drink for women and two drinks for men per day.

- **Estrogen levels.** Low levels of estrogen in postmenopausal women are a significant risk factor for the development of cardiovascular disease in the smaller blood vessels (small vessel heart disease).

Let's take a closer look at estrogen for just a moment, because it has been the subject of much debate and concern among women. When the scientists who were running the Women's Health Initiative (WHI, the largest clinical trial to study the effects of hormone replacement therapy and other factors on heart disease, osteoporosis, and cancer in women) discovered that women who were taking estrogen and progestin had a significantly increased risk of heart attack, stroke, blood clots, and breast cancer, they stopped that part of the study. Then when it was found that women who had had a hysterectomy and who were given only estrogen also had an increased risk of blood clots, stroke, and heart attack, that part of the study was stopped as well.

Because of these findings concerning the impact of estrogen and progestin on the heart, the American Heart Association and the Food and Drug Administration developed new guidelines for the use of hormone replacement therapy. They are:

- Hormone replacement therapy should not be prescribed to prevent heart attack or stroke.

- Use of hormone replacement therapy to prevent osteoporosis should be considered carefully and the risks should be weighed against the benefits. Women who have coronary artery disease should consider other options.

- Hormone replacement therapy may be used for short-term treatment of menopausal symptoms. However, long-term use is discouraged because the risk for heart attack, blood clots, stroke, and breast cancer increases the longer the hormones are taken.

CHAPTER 2

Diagnosing and Treating Heart Disease:
What You Need to Know

Heart disease is the number one killer in the United States, yet many people know very little about how it is diagnosed, when they should be screened, which screening techniques are available, and what their treatment options are once heart disease has been uncovered.

In the first chapter we talked about the risk factors for heart disease, but now it's time to take the next step. We believe it is important for you to have some basic information about the screening, diagnostic, and treatment options for heart disease at your disposal. Chances are very good that you or someone you know and love will be diagnosed with heart disease. As an informed health-care consumer, you can be better prepared to deal with the many questions and decisions that you may need to make.

Therefore, in this chapter we explore two main areas:

- Screening and diagnostic tests and procedures that are used to detect and diagnose heart disease, which include but are not limited to blood tests for levels of homocysteine, cholesterol,

C-reactive protein, and fibrinogen; electrocardio-gram, stress test, echocardiogram, and cardiac catheterization; and

• Medical management of heart disease, including prescription medications, corrective procedures, and surgery, as well as complementary treatment options.

SCREENING FOR HEART DISEASE

In 2002, the American Heart Association (AHA) updated its guidelines on how to prevent heart disease and stroke. The AHA took this step partly because cardiovascular disease continues to be the leading cause of death in the United States, and more and more young people are developing the risk factors for these deadly diseases at an earlier age. Because heart disease and stroke are preventable and risk factors can be minimized through changes in lifestyle, an understanding of screening and early detection is critical.

That said, the AHA recommends that adults begin screening for risk factors as early as age 20 and, by age 40, they should know their absolute risk of developing heart disease. Although the risk factor assessment list given below is a guideline for physicians to implement with their patients, the AHA emphasizes that individuals—you— are the critical element in any successful prevention plan. The AHA hopes men and women will take the initiative and be screened for cardiovascular disease and follow the recommended lifestyle changes that can result in better health and a longer life.

The AHA risk factor assessment list recommended for your physician includes:

- Update regularly: family history

- At every routine evaluation: doctor should ask about smoking status, diet, alcohol intake, physical activity

- At each visit, at least every two years: doctor should measure blood pressure, body mass index, waist circumference, pulse

- At least every 5 years, every 2 years if risk factors are present: doctor should test for fasting serum lipoprotein (lipid profile) or total and HDL cholesterol, and fasting blood glucose

Now let's look at some of the screening procedures included in the risk factor assessment list. The lifestyle risk factors—smoking, diet, alcohol, physical activity—are discussed in detail in chapter 3 on prevention.

Blood Pressure and Pulse

Blood pressure is the pressure the blood exerts against the walls of the arteries. When your doctor gives you your blood pressure result, the top number is the systolic figure, which represents the pressure while the heart contracts to pump blood through the body. The bottom number is the diastolic figure, which represents the pressure when the heart relaxes between beats.

Where does your blood pressure reading fall?

- Less than 120/80 mmHg: Optimal for adults

- 120 to 139 mmHg over 80 to 89 mmHg: Prehypertension, which means you should be implementing positive lifestyle changes to prevent any further increase and bring your blood pressure down

- 140 and greater over 90 or greater: Elevated blood pressure, which means it's time to seriously implement lifestyle changes and talk to your doctor about possibly using medications if lifestyle changes do not give you the results you need.

Body Mass Index

The body mass index (BMI) is a measure of body fat based on weight and height. It is used for both adult men and women and is a reliable indicator of body fat. Although BMI does not measure body fat directly, research shows that BMI correlates to more direct measures, such as underwater weighing.

BMI is a screening and not a diagnostic tool. Your doctor can use your BMI along with other assessments to determine your risk of heart disease. BMI is often used because it is convenient, inexpensive, and easy to use, even by the general public.

To determine your BMI, multiply your weight in pounds by 703, divide by your height in inches, then divide once more by your height in inches.

Generally, the categories are as follows:

- Underweight: <18.5 BMI

- Normal weight: 18.5–24.9

- Overweight: 25.0–29.9

- Obese: 30.0 or greater

Waist Circumference

Your waist circumference is associated with an increased risk for hypertension, cardiovascular disease, type 2 diabetes, and high cholesterol when your body mass index (BMI) is between 25 and 34.9, according to the National Institutes of Health. Changes in your waist circumference over time can indicate an increase or decrease in the amount of abdominal fat you are carrying. Increased abdominal fat is associated with an increased risk of heart disease.

You don't need your doctor to determine your waist circumference. Using a measuring tape, locate your upper hip bone and place the tape around your abdomen. Keep the tape snug but not tight.

You need to know your body mass index and waist circumference to determine your overall risk for the health conditions mentioned. You can use the chart below as a guide.

BMI	Waist Circumference <or= 40" Male, 35" female	Waist Circumference >or= 40" male, 35" female
25.0–29.9	Increased	High
30.0–34.9	High	Very High
35.0–39.9	Very High	Very High
40.0 or greater	Extremely high	Extremely high

Total Cholesterol

A total cholesterol test provides a rough measure of all the cholesterol and triglycerides in your blood. It is part of a lipid panel, which also includes low-density lipoprotein (LDL) cholesterol, high-density lipoprotein (HDL) cholesterol, and triglycerides. If your total cholesterol level is high, your doctor may order a lipid panel (see below). Children who are at high risk of heart disease (i.e., they have some of the same risk factors as adults do for heart disease, including hypertension, obesity, and family history) should undergo their first lipid panel between the ages of two and 10 years, according to the American Academy of Pediatrics.

A total cholesterol test requires that you fast from food and beverages for eight to 12 hours before having your blood drawn. Water is the only item you are allowed to consume during fasting. If you take medications, you need to talk to your doctor about what you can take during a fast.

When you get your total cholesterol reading, see where it falls in these guidelines.

• Desirable: less than 200 mg/dL

• Borderline high cholesterol: 200 to 239 mg/dL

• High risk: 240 mg/dL and higher

Generally, a total cholesterol reading greater than 200 mg/dL means you have an increased risk of heart disease. However, LDL levels are a better predictor of heart disease, and other factors should also be considered, such as C-reactive protein, homocysteine, and waist circumference. However, a reading of 200 mg/dL or higher means it's time to implement some positive lifestyle changes, especially regarding your diet. The foods and supplements covered in chapters 4 and 5 of this book are a great place to start.

Lipid Profile (Fasting Serum Lipoprotein)

A lipid profile is a group of tests that are usually ordered together to determine risk of coronary heart disease. These tests are good indicators of whether individuals are likely to have a stroke or heart attack. A lipid profile includes figures for total cholesterol, HDL cholesterol, LDL cholesterol, and triglycerides. Like the total cholesterol test, it involves a simple blood draw, which can be done at a clinic, hospital, or doctor's office.

When you get your test results back, you can use the following chart to see where your levels are. You and your doctor should discuss the results and what, if any, action needs to be taken to improve your results. The National Cholesterol Education Program, the American Heart Association, and the American College of Cardiology recommend lifestyle changes (e.g., diet, stress management, smoking, exercise) as the first line of defense against abnormal lipid levels. This book is a great place to start with the dietary changes!

Element	Optimal	Borderline	High Risk
LDL cholesterol	<100	130–159	160+
HDL cholesterol	>60	35–45	<35
Triglycerides	<150	150–199	>200
Total cholesterol	<200	200–239	>240

Fasting Blood Glucose

A fasting blood glucose test measures the amount of glucose (sugar) in your blood after you have fasted for at least eight hours. It is a screening test for diabetes and for people at risk of heart disease, as diabetes and heart disease often appear together.

When you get your test results, they will be compared against the normal levels for fasting glucose, which is less than 100 mg/dL (100 milligrams of glucose for each deciliter of blood). If your results are 100 to 125 mg/dL, your doctor will likely recommend that you take another blood test to confirm the first results. If your blood glucose measures 126 mg/dL or higher, your doctor will order a second test. If the results are 126 mg/dL or higher again, you will be diagnosed with diabetes.

DIAGNOSTIC TESTS FOR HEART DISEASE

Depending on the results of your screening tests, your doctor may then order diagnostic tests for heart disease. Below is an explanation of some of the diagnostic tests your doctor may order. Typically the results of no one test alone are used to make a diagnosis, which is why your doctor will likely order several tests.

Homocysteine Test

Homocysteine is made naturally in the body and is a metabolite of the amino acid methionine. Abnormally high levels of homocysteine are associated with a high risk for heart attack or stroke, as this amino acid can damage blood vessels. A homocysteine test may be helpful for patients who have a family history of coronary artery disease but no other risk factors. A growing number of doctors are using the homocysteine test as part of their diagnostic process, but it is not yet recommended by the AHA as part of a routine diagnostic process. Doctors may order a homocysteine test as part of a cardiac risk assessment, or following a stroke or heart attack to help determine a treatment program.

High levels of homocysteine (greater than 16 umol/L) can be caused by insufficient levels of folic acid, vitamin B_6, and/or vitamin B_{12} in your diet; kidney disease; Alzheimer's disease; excessive alcohol use; and certain cancers. For many people, homocysteine levels can be decreased by taking extra amounts of folic acid, vitamin B_6, and vitamin B_{12}.

C-Reactive Protein Test

C-reactive protein (CRP) is a protein in the blood whose levels rise when inflammation is present in the body. A CRP test is used to screen for inflammatory conditions, but a more sensitive CRP test, called high-sensitivity CRP (hs-CRP), can screen for coronary heart disease and cardiovascular disease. An hs-CRP is usually ordered as one of several tests when a doctor is doing a cardiovascular risk profile, usually with tests for cholesterol and triglycerides.

The American Heart Association and the U.S. Centers for Disease Control and Prevention have determined the risk of heart disease associated with the following CRP values (measured in milligrams per liter).

- Low risk: less than 1.0 mg/L

- Average risk: 1.0 to 3.0 mg/L

- High risk: greater than 3.0 mg/L

People who have values in the high end of the normal range have one and a half to four times the risk of experiencing a heart attack as those with hs-CRP values at the low end of the normal range.

Fibrinogen Test

Fibrinogen is a sticky, fibrous protein that plays a key role in blood clotting. A fibrinogen test may be ordered to help your doctor evaluate your body's ability to form a blood clot. The test may be ordered, along with other cardiac risk tests such as CRP, to determine a patient's overall risk of developing cardiovascular disease. Although the test is not widely used, some doctors believe it gives them important information that can help them in treating their patients.

For example, fibrinogen concentrations may rise sharply in people who have an inflammatory condition or tissue damage. Thus elevated levels may be seen in people who have coronary heart disease, myocardial infarction, and stroke.

Electrocardiogram

An electrocardiogram, also known as EKG or ECG, measures the electrical activity of the heartbeat. Every time your heart beats, an electrical wave passes through the heart. The wave causes the muscle to squeeze and pump blood from the heart.

An EKG provides two main types of information. One, it tells clinicians how long the electrical wave takes to pass through the heart. This lets the clinicians know if the electrical activity is normal or slow, fast, or irregular. Two, by measuring the amount of electrical activity that passes through the heart, a cardiologist may determine if parts of the heart are damaged or overworked.

An EKG is a painless procedure that involves placing stickers with leads on your chest and several other locations. The EKG machine does not cause any sensation while it takes its readings.

Stress Test

A stress test, also referred to as a treadmill or exercise test, provides information about how well the heart handles stress (work). As your body works harder during the test, the heart must pump more blood to deliver more oxygen to the body. An exercise stress test can indicate if the blood supply in the arteries is reduced and the kind and degree of exercise that is appropriate for the patient.

During a typical stress test, you will be hooked up to heart monitoring equipment and then begin to walk slowly on a treadmill. The speed and incline on the treadmill will be gradually increased, and you will be asked to breathe into a tube to measure respirations. The technician will monitor heart rate, breathing, blood pressure, fatigue level, and electrocardiogram during the test. You can stop the test at any time if you feel too breathless or ill. When the exercise test is over (it usually takes about 15 to 20 minutes), you will sit or lie down and have your heart rate and blood pressure checked.

A health-care professional may recommend an exercise stress test to:

- Diagnose coronary artery disease

- Predict the risk of heart-related conditions such as heart attack

- Diagnose the cause of heart-related symptoms

such as shortness of breath, lightheadedness, chest pain, and leg pain

• Identify a safe level of exercise for a patient

• Monitor the effectiveness of procedures performed to improve coronary artery blood circulation in patients who have coronary artery disease

Based on the results of the exercise stress test, your doctor may order other tests such as cardiac catheterization.

Echocardiogram

An echocardiogram is a noninvasive test that uses sound waves to create a moving picture of the heart in real time. The test is done to evaluate the valves and chambers of the heart and allows clinicians to check the heart's pumping function, evaluate heart murmurs, and monitor patients who have had a heart attack.

The test is done by a technician who places a device called a transducer on the ribs near the breastbone. The transducer detects the echoes of the sound waves and transmits them as electrical impulses, and the echocardiography machine translates these impulses into moving pictures of the heart.

An abnormal echocardiogram can indicate many different conditions, some of which are very minor, while others are signs of serious heart disease. Therefore it is important that you discuss the results with your health-care provider.

Cardiac Catheterization

A cardiac catheterization is an invasive procedure that allows clinicians to examine blood flow to the heart and test how well the heart is pumping. A doctor inserts a catheter (thin plastic tube) into an artery or vein in the leg or arm and advances the tube into the coronary arteries or the chambers of the heart. The test can measure blood pressure within the heart and how much oxygen is in the blood.

If a dye is injected into the arteries, the procedure is called a coronary angiography. The dye can show whether plaque has accumulated in any of the coronary arteries and is restricting blood flow, which can lead to coronary heart disease. Doctors can take blood and heart muscle samples during cardiac catheterization and also conduct minor heart surgery.

Cardiac catheterization is usually performed in a hospital. Patients are awake during the procedure, and it typically causes little or no pain. Many patients experience some soreness in the blood vessel where the catheter is inserted.

TREATMENT OF HEART DISEASE

Treatment of heart disease can include medication, procedures, surgery, and complementary therapies. In this section we explore some of the more common options in each category.

Medications

If you have been diagnosed with heart disease, you may be surprised at the vast number of medications that are available for treatment. Your doctor may prescribe a variety of drugs designed to address various symptoms, such as high blood pressure, high cholesterol, accumulation of fluids, and chest pain.

No two treatment plans for heart disease are alike: Your doctor will determine which medications and complementary treatments fit your specific symptoms and meet your overall health needs. To prepare your treatment plan, your doctor can choose from drugs in many different categories. Below is a summary of the different categories and what the drugs in each are designed to do.

Ace Inhibitors. Angiotensin converting enzyme (ACE) inhibitors dilate or widen blood vessels to improve blood flow, increase the amount of blood the heart pumps, and lower blood pressure. Doctors may prescribe ACE inhibitors to treat high blood pressure, heart failure, heart attack, and diabetes. They are also prescribed to help decrease the risk of having a heart attack or stroke in high-risk individuals. Examples of ACE inhibitors include captopril (Capoten), lisinopril (Zestril), and enalapril (Vasotec).

Angiotensin II receptor blockers. These drugs, called ARBs for short, are similar to ACE inhibitors, but they work by a different mechanism. ARBs decrease the amount of certain chemicals that cause blood vessels to narrow, which then allows blood to flow easier. They also reduce the amount of certain chemicals that cause fluids to accumulate in the body. Examples of ARBs include losartan (Cozaar), valsartan (Diovan), and telmisartan (Micardis).

Antiarrhythmia drugs. Abnormal heart rhythms, which result from irregular electrical activity in the heart, are treated with antiarrhythmia drugs. Examples include amiodarone (Cordarone), solalol (Betapace), and procainamide (Procanbid).

Antiplatelets. Antiplatelet drugs prevent the formation of blood clots. Platelets can accumulate when a blood vessel is damaged, as occurs during atherosclerosis. Antiplatelet drugs can prevent the formation of blood clots, which can lead to heart attack or stroke. Doctors may prescribe antiplatelets for patients who have a history of coronary artery disease, heart attack, angina, stroke, and peripheral artery disease.

Beta-blockers. This group of drugs relax the heart, reduce the production of harmful substances the body produces in response to heart failure, and slow the heart rate. They are often prescribed to treat angina, heart failure, high blood pressure, abnormal heart rhythms, and heart attack. Examples of beta-blockers include atenolol (Tenormin), metoprolol (Lopressor), and propranolol (Inderal).

Calcium channel blockers. These drugs relax blood vessels and increase the supply of oxygen and blood to the heart. Calcium channel blockers are often prescribed for coronary artery disease, coronary spasm, angina, abnormal heart rhythms, hypertrophic cardiomyopathy, and diastolic heart failure. Examples of calcium channel blockers include amlodipine (Norvasc), diltiazem (Cardizem), and nicardipine (Cardene).

Digoxin. This medication helps a heart that has been injured or weakend to work more efficiently by slowing the heart rate, improving blood circulation, and improving the heart's contractions. Doctors prescribed digoxin to treat atrial fibrillation and heart failure. Digoxin is sold under several trade names (e.g., Lanoxin, Lanoxicaps).

Diuretics. Also known as water pills, diuretics help the body eliminate excess water and salt through the urine, which reduces blood pressure and makes it easier for the heart to pump. Diuretics are categorized as thiazide-like, loop, and potassium-sparing. Thiazide diuretics are appropriate for long-term use, loop diuretics are more potent and best for emergencies, and potassium-sparing diuretics help the body keep potassium. They are often prescribed along with the other two types of diuretics. Diuretics are typically prescribed to treat edema, high blood pressure, heart failure, and kidney problems. Examples of diuretics include bumetanide (Bumex), furosemide (Lasix), and spironolactone (Aldactone).

Inotropics. These medications are only prescribed when other drugs have failed to control heart failure symptoms. Inotropics stimulate a weak or injured heart to pump harder. Examples include dobutaine (Dobutrex) and milrinone (Primacor).

Thrombolytics. Also known as clot busters, these drugs are given in the hospital intravenously to break up blood clots. Typically they are administered to prevent the ongoing damage of heart attacks, to prevent ongoing damage from ischemic stroke, and to break up blood clots in other blood vessels in the body. Examples of thrombolytics include tissue plasminogen activator (TPA), alteplase, and streptokinase.

Vasodilators. People who have heart failure or high blood pressure may be prescribed vasodilators. These drugs relax the blood vessels to allow blood to flow more easily. Doctors may recommend vasodilators for patients who cannot take ACE inhibitors or angiotensin receptor blockers. Examples of vasodilators include isosorbide dinitrate (Dilatrate, Isordil), hydralazine (Apresoline), and isorbide mononitrate (IMDUR).

Warfarin. This anticoagulant medication helps prevent clots from forming. This blood thinner (trade name Coumadin) is used to treat various types of heart disease, and is often prescribed for atrial fibrillation, pulmonary embolism, and after artificial heart valve surgery.

Procedures and Surgeries

When medication, lifestyle changes, and/or complementary therapies are not enough to reduce symptoms or repair or restore heart function, medical procedures or surgery may be necessary. Surgery is often recommended for patients who have unstable angina that has not responded to medical treatment, severe recurrent episodes of angina that last more than 20 minutes, or those who have severe coronary artery disease (e.g., severe angina, multi-artery involvement, evidence of ischemia). It is recommended that you learn all you can about any procedure or surgery your doctor may recommend, and you should also get a second opinion.

Here are some of the more common procedures and surgeries associated with heart disease. We begin with the procedures.

Angioplasty and stents. Angioplasty is a nonsurgical technique that is performed to open a blocked artery. You are awake during the procedure, but well medicated so you can relax. During angioplasty, a catheter is inserted into an artery. Contrast material is injected through the catheter and photographed so the clinician can see whether the arteries are blocked and/or if the heart valves are working properly. If the artery is blocked, the doctor will perform one of various procedures, such as inserting a stent (a tube that helps keep the artery open) or balloon angioplasty (use of a tiny balloon inserted through the catheter to open up the artery). The entire procedure takes about one and a half to two and a half hours, and recovery time is several hours or overnight in the hospital.

Cardioversion. This noninvasive procedure is used to treat heart rhythms that are irregular (arrhythmia). Cardioversion involves use of a special machine that sends electrical energy to the heart muscle to restore normal rhythm. It is often used to treat atrial fibrillation or atrial flutter, but it can also be used to treat ventricular tachycardia. Patients are sedated during the procedure so they don't feel the electrical shocks. If this procedure sounds like defibrillation, you're right, as both involve using a device to deliver electrical shock to the heart. Cardioversion, however, uses much lower electricity levels and it is used in nonemergency situations. Defibrillation is typically used to treat arrhythmias that are difficult to treat, and usually in an emergency.

Bypass surgery. Also called coronary artery bypass graft, it is a very serious but common operation. It involves removing or redirecting a blood vessel from one part of the body (usually the legs, arms, or chest) and placing it around the area that has narrowed in the heart. This blood vessel is called a graft, and it is common for surgeons to bypass three or four coronary arteries during surgery. Bypass surgery can be performed traditionally (requires a six- to eight-inch incision in the chest) or using minimally invasive procedures (a three-inch incision). Not all heart patients are candidates for minimally invasive surgery, but it is an option you should explore with your surgeon.

Heart valve surgery. Heart valve surgery may involve either repairing or replacing a valve. The mitral valve is the most commonly repaired heart valve; the aortic, pulmonic, and tricuspid valves also can be repaired. Several different repair procedures can be performed, depending on the type of damage to the valve. Advantages of valve repair include a decreased need for life-long blood thinning medication, and preserved heart muscle strength. Valves that are too damaged to be repaired can be replaced.

New valves can be donated from a human heart, made of animal tissue (biological valves), or mechanical and made of carbon. Donated valves are preferred, but they are usually in short supply. Recently biological valves have been made that last much longer than their predecessors, at least seventeen years without loss of function, while mechanical valves can last a lifetime if anticoagulant medication is well controlled.

Transmyocardial laser revascularization. This is a new high-tech procedure used to treat inoperable heart disease in people who have persistent angina that has not responded to other methods. Transmyocardial laser revascularization (TMR) is a surgical procedure that improves blood flow to areas of the heart that were not treated previously by surgery or angioplasty. It is performed through a small incision in the left side of the chest and involves using a carbon dioxide laser to create small pathways in the heart to promote blood flow. The laser beams are directed by computer. TMR is an option for patients who have severe angina, evidence of ischemia, a history of previous bypass surgery or angioplasty and no further procedure is available, or those who have been told there is nothing else that can help their symptoms.

Pacemaker. When a heart does not beat regularly, a pacemaker can correct the problem. Pacemakers are usually prescribed to treat bradyarrhythmias (slow heart rhythms), heart failure, fainting spells, and hypertrophic cardiomyopathy. A pacemaker is a small device that is implanted just under the skin of the chest. It typically consists of a pulse generator, which holds the computer and battery, and the leads, which are wires that are threaded through the veins into the heart and implanted into the heart muscle. There are different types of pacemakers—single chamber, dual chamber, and biventricular—and your doctor will determine which type best fits your needs.

Implantable cardioverter defibrillator. An implantable cardioverter defibrillator (ICD) is an electronic device that constantly monitors your heart rate and rhythm and sends energy to the heart when it detects an abnormal rhythm. Similar to a pacemaker, an ICD consists of tiny computer, battery, and leads, and comes in three types: single chamber, dual chamber, and biventricular. It is usually prescribed for people who have had a heart attack or an episode of sudden cardiac arrest or ventricular fibrillation; those who have hypertrophic cardiomyopathy and are at high risk for sudden arrest; and people who have had at least one episode of ventricular tachycardia.

COMPLEMENTARY TREATMENT OPTIONS

In addition to conventional medical approaches to heart disease prevention and treatment, many people are looking for and using complementary therapies. These consist mainly of lifestyle options, such as a regular exercise program, stress management techniques, and dietary and natural supplements. These options are also critical preventive approaches, and so we discuss them in detail in the next chapter. In addition, you can explore the dietary and natural supplement options in our comprehensive coverage of 40 heart-healthy foods and 12 heart-healthy supplements in chapters 4 and 5, respectively, and learn how adding these selections to your life may improve not only your heart but your quality of life as well.

CHAPTER 3

You Can Prevent Heart Disease

Perhaps the best news about heart disease is that you can prevent it. That's because, in most cases, heart disease is the result of poor lifestyle habits—smoking, excessive alcohol use, poor diet, overweight, poor stress management, lack of exercise, and illicit drug use. It is true that genetics can play a part in the development of heart disease, and some people do have congenital heart conditions, as we mentioned in chapter 1. Even in such cases, however, you can make prudent lifestyle choices that can reduce or minimize the impact of those genetic conditions.

So in this chapter we talk about the lifestyle choices you can make that can help you prevent heart disease. You should know that you can make an incredibly powerful difference in your life and in the lives of your family and other loved ones if you decide to make such choices. And one of the great benefits of choosing heart-healthy habits is that they are synergistic.

For example, to prevent heart disease it is important to prevent and control high blood cholesterol and high blood pressure. Both of these health concerns can be prevented and managed by adopting the same heart-healthy habits: eating a healthy diet that is low in saturated fat, getting regular exercise, and maintaining a healthy weight. By adopting a few heart-friendly habits, you can slay several heart-damaging dragons at the same time. It's up to you.

DON'T SMOKE

Smoking cigarettes or cigars or using other tobacco products is a very significant risk factor for the development of heart disease. Exposure to secondhand smoke is also a factor to be considered. What makes smoke and smoking so dangerous?

Nicotine leads to acute increases in blood pressure and heart rate and makes your heart work harder. The carbon monoxide in cigarette smoke replaces some of the oxygen in your blood, which increases blood pressure. Smoking increases blood clotting and also damages the endothelium, which is the layer of cells that lines the blood vessels. It makes the arteries and other blood vessels more vulnerable to narrowing, which can ultimately lead to a heart attack.

Women who smoke and who also take birth control pills are at greater risk of having a stroke or heart attack than women who don't smoke or take the pills. The risk of experiencing either condition increases with age, especially after age 35.

Exposure to secondhand smoke is also harmful to the heart. Environmental tobacco smoke contains more than 4,000 chemicals and at least 40 known carcinogens. A landmark 10-year study (*Circulation* 1997) of more than 32,000 women found that constant exposure to secondhand smoke nearly doubles the risk of having a heart attack.

If you smoke now and you quit, will you reap many benefits? Absolutely. Within just one year of quitting, your risk of heart disease declines dramatically. According to the American Lung Association, within one year of quitting, your excess risk of coronary heart disease is decreased to half that of a smoker. After five years, your stroke risk is reduced to that of people who never smoked. At fifteen years, your risk of coronary heart disease is similar to people who never smoked, and the risk of death returns to nearly the same as people who never smoked.

MOVE, MOVE REGULARLY, HAVE FUN

Move. Move regularly. Have fun. There's no getting around it: you need regular moderately vigorous physical activity to stay healthy, and especially to reduce your risk of heart disease. Experts have noted that inactivity imposes a similar relative risk of heart disease as does high blood pressure, high cholesterol, and smoking. Clearly, being a couch potato is dangerous to your health!

The standard recommendation is to get at least 30 to 60 minutes of moderately intense exercise at least four days per week. If you can't spare 30 minutes at one time, break your activity into two 15- or 20-minute sessions. If you are a very busy person, make a date with yourself each day and write it into your datebook: brisk walk at 7 a.m. for 20 minutes and before lunch for 20 minutes. You know you can do it.

Try some variety: walk the dog (or your neighbor's dog), take the stairs, drop in on an aerobics class occasionally, jog with a friend, ride a bike, go canoeing on the weekend. Just keep moving, move often, and have fun.

EAT TO SAVE YOUR HEART

There are literally hundreds, perhaps thousands of different diets and dietary fads on the market, but the basic eating plan to protect your heart—and for overall health as well—is to eat foods low in fat, cholesterol, and salt; to include lots of fruits, vegetables, and whole grains; and to choose low-fat protein sources such as legumes, certain fish, and low-fat dairy products.

What About Fat?

It's important to watch the types of fat in your diet. Saturated and trans fat increase the risk of coronary artery disease by raising blood cholesterol levels. Saturated fat is found in meat, dairy products (choose low-fat), and coconut and palm oils. Trans fat is found in many processed foods, such as baked goods, crackers, frozen dinners, snack foods, some margarines, and deep-fried fast foods. Trans fat poses an even more significant risk for heart disease because unlike saturated fat, it raises LDL (bad) cholesterol and lowers HDL (good) cholesterol.

Another kind of fat is polyunsaturated fat, and in this category are omega-3 fatty acids, which may decrease the risk of heart attack, lower blood pressure, and protect against arrhythmia. Omega-3 fatty acids can be found in certain fish, including salmon, tuna, and herring, as well as flaxseed oil, walnut oil, and supplements. You can read about several of these foods and supplements in chapters 4 and 5.

What About Vitamin, Minerals, and Other Nutrients?

A big part of a heart-healthy diet can be found in two categories: fruits and vegetables, and whole grains and beans. When you turn to chapter 4, you will see that a large number of the 40 most heart-healthy foods fall into these categories because they are excellent sources of the nutrients—vitamins, minerals, and phytonutrients—that keep the heart and circulatory system going strong. These nutrients are so important for a healthy heart, in fact, that we present a list of them below so you can learn more about these critical substances in your food.

B-complex vitamins: Typically eight vitamins are included in this category: thiamin (B_1), riboflavin (B_2), niacin (B_3), pantothenic acid (B_5), pyridoxine (B_6), folic acid (B_9), and cyanocobalamin (B_{12}). All of the B vitamins benefit the heart and cardiovascular system in some way. For example, vitamin B_6 protects against blood clots and atherosclerosis; niacin helps increase levels of "good" cholesterol; and folic acid is important in the production of red blood cells.

Carotenoids: These heart-protective antioxidants are the pigments that color fruits and vegetables. They include alpha-carotene, beta-carotene, lutein, and lycopene.

Ellagic acid: This acid is a type of polyphenol that is often referred to as a nonflavonoid. It is found in berries (especially red raspberries), walnuts, pecans, tea, and pomegranates.

Flavonoids: These plant substances are a type of polyphenol and include catechins, flavonones, flavonols, isoflavones, reservatrol, and anthocyanins.

Lignans: These are chemical compounds found in the cell walls of plants. Flax and flaxseeds are especially rich in lignans, which are a type of phytoestrogen.

Omega-3 fatty acids: These heart-healthy fatty acids are found in fatty fish, such as salmon and tuna, and in nuts, such as walnuts. They can help boost the immune system, reduce the risk of blood clots, increase high-density lipoprotein (HDL) levels, reduce triglyceride levels, protect against buildup of plaque in the arteries, reduce blood pressure, and fight inflammation.

Phenols: Also known as phenolics, these substances act as antioxidants, prevent blood clots, and prevent inflammation. They can be found in nearly all fruits, vegetables, and grains in varying amounts. Also see *polyphenols*.

Phytoestrogens: Substances in plants that have a weak estrogen-like effect on the body. Flaxseed is a rich source of phytoestrogens, which have been found to reduce the risk of stroke, blood clots, and cardiac arrhythmias, as well as lower blood pressure and triglyceride levels.

Phytonutrients: The term "phytonutrients" is a general term that describes non-vitamin, non-mineral organic substances that are found in plants. Some of the more common phytonutrients we discuss in this book are carotenoids, flavonoids, indoles, nonflavonoids, phenols, saponins, and sulfides.

Phytosterols: These plant sterols are chemically similar to cholesterol and have the ability to reduce blood cholesterol levels. Phytosterols are found in seeds and nuts, including wheat germ.

Polyphenols: These antioxidants can help reduce blood pressure and LDI cholesterol levels and protect the blood vessels. Two types of polyphenols include flavonoids and nonflavonoids.

Saponins: These phytonutrients help block the absorption of cholesterol and thus reduce the amount of fats that circulates in the bloodstream. They are found in tomatoes, garlic, onions, and spinach.

Sulfides: These phytonutrients have the ability to enhance blood circulation and may help lower cholesterol. They are found in sulfur-containing plants such as garlic, chives, leeks, and onions.

Once we leave the produce aisle, we venture into the fish department, where we can find rich sources of omega-3 fatty acids; and we search out various nuts, beans, yogurt, and yes, don't forget the chocolate and red wine! All of these foods and more, plus the 12 heart-healthy supplements discussed in chapter 5, can help prevent heart disease and the complications that are associated with it.

Did Someone Say Fiber?

Fiber is one of the most important dietary factors in a heart-healthy diet, because it helps reduce cholesterol, maintain weight, and keep blood glucose levels in check. Fiber comes in two main forms, soluble and insoluble. The body cannot digest either form, so they are not absorbed into the bloodstream and are eliminated from the body.

Soluble fiber attracts water and turns to gel during digestion. This transformation slows the digestive process and reduces the absorption of cholesterol in the intestines. Studies show that eating 10 grams or more of soluble fiber per day decreases total and LDL cholesterol levels, which in turn reduces your risk of heart disease. One bowl (one and a half cups) of oatmeal alone contains about 6 grams of fiber. Soluble fiber can also help reduce blood sugar levels, which helps in the management of diabetes and thus reduces the associated risk for heart disease. Good sources of soluble fiber include barley, nuts, beans, lentils, and many fruits and vegetables. You can read about the many fiber-rich foods in chapter 4.

Insoluble fiber, while not directly heart-healthy, is important because it aids the digestive process, helps prevent constipation, and promotes regularity. This form of fiber is found in whole grains and many vegetables.

May I Have a Drink?

Numerous studies have shown that drinking alcohol in moderation—no more than two drinks per day for men and one per day for women—can be part of a heart-healthy diet. That doesn't mean you should start drinking if you don't already. But if you do drink wine, beer, or spirits, adhering to the recommended daily intake may prove beneficial for your heart. One drink of each type of alcohol equals the following:

- 5 ounces of wine

- 12 ounces of beer

- 1.5 ounces of 80-proof spirits

- 8 ounces of malt liquor

WATCHING YOUR WEIGHT

One of the realities of life is that as people get older, they tend to gain weight, often a little at a time, just a few pounds per year. One reason for the weight gain is that metabolism usually slows as we age; another reason is that many people become less active and/or eat more. This dangerous combination results in an increase in weight that is mostly fat rather than muscle. In many cases much of the weight gathers around the waist and hips, which increases the risk of heart disease. That's one reason why waist circumference, which we discussed in chapter 2 as part of screening for heart disease, is so important.

You can see if you are at a healthy weight by calculating your body mass index (BMI), which we discussed in chapter 2. The BMI helps you determine whether you are carrying a healthy or unhealthy percentage of body fat.

A recent study (July 2009) demonstrates just how important a healthy weight is for preventing heart disease. Researchers followed 20,525 nonsmoking, nondiabetic, normal-weight men for 7.7 years to assess optimal body weight with respect to minimizing the risk of coronary heart disease. They found that compared to men who had a BMI between 22.5 and 25.0, those who had a BMI less than 22.5 had a 24.1 percent lower risk of coronary heart disease, a 27.9 percent lower risk of nonfatal coronary heart disease, and a 37.8 percent lower risk of nonfatal myocardial infarction. The researchers concluded that the optimal BMI for minimizing your risk of coronary heart disease is less than 22.5.

Studies also show that even small amounts of weight loss can help your heart. If you reduce your weight by just 10 percent (that's 20 pounds for a 200-pound person), you can lower your blood pressure, reduce your cholesterol levels, and lower your risk of diabetes—all significant risk factors for heart disease.

GET REGULAR HEALTH SCREENINGS

We cannot stress the importance of this preventive measure enough. Why? Many people, for example, are unaware that they have high blood pressure and/or high cholesterol because both of these conditions typically have no symptoms. That means both hypertension and high cholesterol can seriously damage your heart and blood vessels without your knowledge, and your first wake-up call may be a heart attack or stroke.

To prevent these unwelcome events, regular screenings are recommended, as we discussed in chapter 2. Regular blood pressure screenings should begin in childhood, especially if a child is overweight or has a family history of high blood pressure. Adults should be screened for blood pressure at least every two years. You should be screened more often if any of your readings are not optimal (less than 120/80 mmHg) and/or if you have other risk factors for heart disease.

Screening for cholesterol levels also should be done in adults at least once every five years. If your cholesterol levels are not optimal (200 mg/dL or lower) and/or if you have other risk factors for heart disease, you should have a cholesterol test more frequently. Children should be screened for cholesterol levels if they have a strong family history of heart disease and/or if they are overweight.

Other screenings as recommended by the American Heart Association are outlined in chapter 2. Remember, heart disease is often avoidable. You have the power to prevent it if you incorporate heart-healthy habits into your life.

PART II

**Foods and Supplements
to Promote a Healthy Heart**

CHAPTER 4

Heart-Healthy Foods: A to Z

Which foods should you include in your daily diet to help protect your heart? That's the question we answer for you in this chapter. We have scoured the popular and scientific literature and come up with a list of the top 40 foods that can promote and maintain the health of your heart and the blood vessels that support it. We provide detailed information and suggestions on easy and delicious ways to prepare each of these foods so you can better appreciate them and how they can make your life better.

Researchers are discovering new information about the intimate relationship between nutrition and the heart all the time, and we believe you should know about it. That's why, along with background information and a recipe for each food item, we include the results of the latest scientific research about a specific food or its heart-healthy components. Did you know, for example, that experts recently found that plums equal or surpass blueberries in antioxidant power? You can read about the power of plums and much more in this chapter.

Each entry in this chapter includes (as appropriate) a

definition of the food, a history of its use, the properties that make it a heart-healthy candidate, the science behind the claims, and a recipe suggestion on how to include the food into your diet. These recipes are the ones we refer to in the seven-day menu in chapter 6.

Before we discuss the foods, however, we want to explain the nutritional value information that you will find in each food entry.

HOW WE CALCULATED
THE NUTRITIONAL VALUES

The percentages given in the nutritional value sections of each entry are based on the Daily Reference Intake (DRI) figures determined by the Food and Nutrition Board, Institutes of Medicine, for male and female adults ages 19 years and older. DRI values are based on the average requirements for males and females of all ages and include Estimated Average Requirements (EAR), Recommended Dietary Allowances (RDA), Tolerable Upper Intake Levels (UL), and Adequate Intake (AI) values.

The recommended values for adult men and women within the same age group are different for some nutrients and the same for others. For consistency, we based our percentage calculations on the higher figure in any given range when a range is given. For example, the DRI values for vitamin C are 75 mg for women and 90 mg for men, so we used the 90 mg figure. Because there is no DRI for fiber, we based our percentage on the average of the recommended range for females (25 grams) and males (38 grams) as 32 grams daily.

Daily Reference Intakes for Adults 19 Years +
(Numbers given are for the higher number in the
range for males and females)

Vitamin A	3,000 IU
Vitamin C	90 mg
Vitamin D	600 IU
Vitamin E	22 IU natural vitamin E; 33 IU synthetic
Thiamin	1.2 mg
Riboflavin	1.3 mg
Niacin	16 mg
B_5	5 mg
B_6	1.7 mg
Folic acid	400 mcg
B_{12}	2.4 mcg
Iron	8.1 mg
Magnesium	420 mg
Manganese	2.3 mg

Potassium	4700 mg
Selenium	55 mcg
Zinc	11 mg

ALMONDS

Are you nuts about nuts? Then almonds are a great choice. Almonds have been considered a healing food since ancient times. The earliest varieties of almonds were transported along the Silk Road from China to the Middle East. During classical Roman times and among the early Europeans, almonds were considered a symbol of fertility. In Sweden today, the almond is a sign of good fortune: if you get the almond hidden in the Christmas pudding, you will have good luck all year long. Today we know almonds are good luck because they are heart-healthy.

NUTRITIONAL INFORMATION—ALMONDS
¼ cup raw
Calories: 205
Protein: 7.6 g
Fiber: 4 g, 13%
Magnesium: 76 mg, 18% DRI
Riboflavin: 0.3 mg, 23% DRI
Vitamin E: 9 mg, 18% DRI

Why Almonds Are Heart-Healthy

Each one-ounce serving of almonds (about 23 nuts) offers a rich source of vitamin E, magnesium, and manganese, and a good source of fiber, copper, riboflavin, and phosphorus, along with 12 grams of heart-healthy unsaturated fats. A 2006 study found that each ounce of almonds contains about the same amount of polyphenols as one cup of green tea and one-half cup of steamed broccoli. The scientists used high-level technology to detect flavonoids and phenolics in the skins of almonds that are similar to those found in certain fruits and vegetables.

More than a dozen studies have shown that almonds have a positive impact on cholesterol levels and on risks for coronary heart disease. In a 2002 study published in *Circulation,* for example, the scientists found that almonds significantly reduced blood lipid levels (e.g., low-density lipoprotein cholesterol, triglycerides), partly because of their monounsaturated fat and fiber content.

Several large studies, including the Nurses Health Study and the Iowa Health Study, found that eating nuts is associated with a reduced risk for heart disease. If you eat just one ounce of almonds daily, you may significantly reduce your total and LDL cholesterol levels by 4 and 5 percent, respectively. The potassium also protects against high blood pressure.

RECIPE
Rather than toasted almonds, why not toast *with* your almonds! Try this tasty almond beverage for a change of pace.

Almond Banana Beverage
Serves 2–3
1 cup raw almonds, no skins
6 cups filtered water
1 small ripe banana
Stevia to taste

Soak the almonds in 3 cups of water in the refrigerator overnight (at least 8 hours). Drain the soaked almonds and process in a blender with 3 cups of fresh filtered water until you get a milky consistency. Strain the mixture through a sprout bag or cheesecloth to remove the almond pulp. (Hint: the almond pulp can be refrigerated and used in cookie recipes that call for almonds or almond paste.) Place the mixture back into the blender and add the banana. Blend until smooth. Add stevia to taste. Keep refrigerated for up to three days in a container with a tight lid.

APPLES

Apples have a long and honored history as a symbol of fertility and love and as an aphrodisiac, the perfect dessert before an evening of romance. The adage about an apple a day keeping the doctor away may have something to do with the fact that apples were associated with the Greek healing god, Apollo, or that Greek doctors living in Rome, including Galen and Hippocrates, recommended eating sweet apples to aid digestion, while suggesting sour apples to treat constipation and fainting. Apple juice also reportedly had medicinal value as an antidepressant.

Remains of apples have been found at archaeological sites, including excavations at Jericho in the Jordan Valley from 500 B.C. Apples have long been a favorite fruit, and their popularity led to experimentation. The first controlled apple hybridization program to improve apples was started in 1790 in England. Since then consumers have hundreds of varieties of apples from which to choose, all nutritious and delicious. There are at least several varieties available at any point throughout the year.

NUTRITIONAL VALUE—APPLES
3 1/4" diameter
Calories: 116
Fiber: 5.4 g, 17%
Vitamin C: 10 mg, 9% DRI

Why Apples Are Heart-Healthy

Apples are blessed with a variety of phytonutrients, including the potent flavonoid quercetin, that are important for heart health. If you want to reap the benefits of quercetin, however, you will need to keep the skin on, as this phytonutrient is found solely in apple skin, not the flesh. Here are some reasons why eating an apple a day may be a great idea.

- A study of more than 34,000 postmenopausal women found that apples are one of three foods (red wine and pears are the other two) that reduce the risk of mortality for both coronary heart disease and cardiovascular disease. Apples are an especially rich source of flavonoids, including quercetin, epicatechin, epigallacatechin, kaempferol, and others. Flavonoids are key for heart health for several reasons. Some help prevent inflammation, others help prevent clumping of blood platelets, and others help regulate blood pressure and overproduction of fat in the liver. The women in the study were part of the ongoing Iowa Women's Health Study, which has been underway for about 20 years. Although women of all ages are encouraged to eat foods high in flavonoids (fruits, vegetables, nuts, tea, seeds), this study, published in the March 2007 *American Journal of Clinical*

Nutrition, focused on postmenopausal women, a population that is at higher risk for heart disease than are younger women.

- Apples are a rich source of pectin, a form of soluble fiber, and insoluble fiber (cellulose). Both types of fiber can help reduce LDL cholesterol levels.

- Apples contain a high amount of antioxidants, which help protect the entire cardiovascular system from free-radical damage to the cells that are responsible for carrying oxygen throughout the body.

RECIPE

This recipe is a great way to start the day, but it can just as well be a dessert or snack.

Baked Apple with Crunch
Serves 2
2 medium apples
¹/₂ cup apple juice
2 Tbs of chopped figs
¹/₄ tsp ground cinnamon
¹/₄ cup low-fat granola cereal
1 Tbs ground flaxseed

Chop the apples into bite-sized pieces (keep the skin on). Mix the apple pieces with the figs and place in a small casserole. Sprinkle with cinnamon and pour the apple juice over the mixture. Cover the casserole and bake in a

350°F oven for 20 minutes. Remove from the oven and top with a mixture of granola and flaxseed. Serve warm.

APRICOTS

The predecessor to the delicate, velvety, and very sweet apricot we are familiar with today was discovered in China about 4,000 years ago. At that time the Chinese came face to face with the wild ancestor to the present day apricot. The Chinese were the first to cultivate the ancient fruit. Tradition says that the Chinese considered the apricot to have fertility-promoting abilities, which may be one reason it grew in popularity. Another reason is likely its sweet flavor and fragrance.

Spanish explorers brought apricots to the New World in the eighteenth century, and the fruit trees landed in California in the gardens of Spanish missions. To this day California is the main home of apricot production in the United States, where more than 95 percent of the crop is grown.

NUTRITIONAL VALUE—APRICOTS, RAW
1 cup slices
Calories: 79
Fiber: 3.3 g, 10%
Vitamin A: 3,178 IU, 106% DRI
Potassium: 427 mg, 9% DRI

NUTRITIONAL VALUE—APRICOTS, DRIED
1 ounce
Calories: 90
Vitamin A: 3,547 IU, 118% DRI

Iron: 1.8 mg, 22% DRI
Potassium: 518 mg, 11% DRI

Why Apricots Are Heart-Healthy

Fresh apricots are a healthy treat, but dried apricots provide even more nutrition. That's because the drying process increases the concentration of the beta-carotene and fiber and also the levels of potassium and iron.

- Apricots contain a good amount of fiber, which helps lower cholesterol levels.

- The high levels of beta-carotene/vitamin A and lycopene in apricots protect low-density lipoprotein (LDL) cholesterol from oxidation, which helps prevent heart disease.

- Getting an adequate amount of potassium is crucial for maintaining a healthy, strong heartbeat. If you have heart failure, heart rhythm problems, or high blood pressure, this mineral is especially important. A diet that is rich in potassium can help lower blood pressure.

- Two separate large studies show the advantage of eating foods rich in beta-carotene, such as apricots. In a Harvard study of 87,000 female nurses, those who ate the most beta-carotene-rich foods (equal to 1.5 carrots daily) had a 22 percent lower risk of heart disease than women who ate the least amount of such foods. In a University of Texas study, men who ate 6 mg of beta-carotene daily (equal to 1 carrot) over 25 years had a 28 percent lower risk of death from all causes.

RECIPE

To get the most nutritional benefits from apricots, eat them raw or dried. Here is a recipe that is good for breakfast or as a snack.

Apricot Hats
12 fresh apricots, halved
4 ounces low-fat cream cheese
1/2 cup finely chopped almonds or walnuts
3 figs, cut into quarters

Stir the cream cheese until it is smooth and stir in the chopped nuts. Spoon the mixture into the center of each apricot half. Top each apricot with a quartered fig.

ASPARAGUS

The ancient Egyptians so revered the asparagus that they cultivated it for medicinal purposes and offered it to their gods. This highly nutritious vegetable, which has also been touted as an aphrodisiac (mainly because of its shape), has been used over the centuries to treat infertility, arthritis, and toothaches, among other ailments. It gained popularity in Europe during the sixteenth century and was first cultivated in the United States beginning in the nineteenth century. Today, asparagus is grown in many countries around the world, with California being the main producer in the United States.

Asparagus is available in green, white, and purple

varieties. Purple asparagus originated in Italy and tends to be sweeter and more tender than the green and white varieties. White asparagus is actually green asparagus. Because the sun turns the emerging stalks green, farmers who want white asparagus heap about six inches of dirt on top of the plants so they will grow underground. When the tip of the asparagus breaks through the soil, workers must use a special knife to cut the white stalks.

NUTRITIONAL VALUE—ASPARAGUS
1 cup cooked, fresh
Calories: 43
Fiber: 2.9 g, 9%
Folic acid: 263 mcg, 66% DRI
Vitamin A: 970 IU, 32% DRI
Vitamin C: 19 mg, 21% DRI
Potassium: 288 mg, 6% DRI

Why Asparagus Is Heart-Healthy
Only 20 of the approximately 300 different varieties of asparagus are edible, and all of them offer a powerful array of nutrients. Here's how they can help your heart.

- The high potassium content in asparagus, along with its low sodium level and the amino acid asparagine, are the ingredients for an effective natural diuretic. Thus asparagus can help with high blood pressure and water retention.

- Elevated levels of a substance called homocysteine significantly increase the risk for heart disease. Approximately 20 to 40 percent of people with heart disease have high homocysteine levels.

Asparagus stalks contain high levels of folic acid, a nutrient (along with vitamin B_6 and B_{12}) known to help reduce homocysteine levels. A good amount of B_6 is also found in asparagus.

- High levels of the antioxidant vitamins A and C are beneficial for the heart. Although studies don't always support the use of antioxidant supplements as a way to help promote heart health, research does show that consuming foods rich in antioxidants is associated with a reduced risk of cardiovascular disease.

- Asparagus contains high levels of rutin, a flavonoid that strengthens capillary walls and that in animal studies has been shown to lower cholesterol.

RECIPE
You can make this recipe with green, white, or purple asparagus—or all three!

Simply Asparagus
Serves 2–4
1 lb asparagus
2 Tbs olive oil
2 Tbs grated Parmesan cheese
2 Tbs almond slivers
1 tsp lemon zest
Salt and black pepper to taste

Cut asparagus into 1- to 2-inch pieces and place in a saucepan that is filled halfway with boiling water. Parboil the asparagus for 2 minutes. Drain off the water and place vegetables in a bowl. Add the remaining ingredients and mix well. Serve warm.

BANANAS

Experts believe that bananas originated in Malaysia about 4,000 years ago and then eventually were carried to India and the Philippines. Arabian traders brought the fruit to Africa, and Portuguese explorers discovered them there in 1482. We can thank the Portuguese for transporting the fruit to the Americas.

Originally only people who lived along the coasts of the United States could enjoy bananas because they were too fragile to transport long distances into the mainland. With the development of refrigeration in the twentieth century, however, they rapidly become popular everywhere. The main commercial growers of bananas today are Costa Rica, Mexico, Ecuador, and Brazil.

NUTRITIONAL VALUE—BANANAS
1 medium: 7"–7 7/8" long
Calories: 105
Fiber: 3.1 g, 10%
Potassium: 422 mg, 9% DRI
Vitamin B_6: 0.43 mg, 25% DRI
Vitamin C: 10 mg, 11% DRI

Why Bananas Are Heart-Healthy

You may already know that bananas are one of the best sources of potassium, which is an essential mineral when it comes to heart health. Studies show that bananas also harbor other nutrients that are beneficial for cardiac health.

To get the most mileage from a banana's antioxidants, eat the fruit when it is fully ripe. To hear what the experts have to say, let's look at some study results.

- The potassium in just one banana—about 460 mg for a medium fruit—and its extremely low sodium level of 1 mg makes it a good candidate to help prevent against high blood pressure and atherosclerosis. In one study, for example, more than 40,000 men were followed for more than four years to identify the impact of diet on their blood pressure. The men who ate the most potassium-rich foods, along with foods high in cereal fiber and magnesium, had a substantially reduced risk of stroke.

- The fiber in bananas helps the heart. In a 2003 study published in the *Archives of Internal Medicine,* the authors reported on nearly 10,000 adults whom they followed for 19 years. They found that people who consumed the most fiber daily (21 grams) has 11 percent less cardiovascular disease and 12 percent less coronary heart disease than the participants who ate the least (5 grams) amount of fiber daily.

- One banana contains about one-third the daily requirement of vitamin B_6, which is essential for helping to eliminate homocysteine, the heart-damaging amino acid. Vitamin B_6 works along with vitamin B_{12} and folic acid to accomplish this task.

RECIPE

Bananas are a fun fruit: easy to carry around, easy to peel, and easy to eat just about any time and anywhere. Although we encourage you to eat fresh, raw bananas any time, sometimes it's fun to shake it up a bit.

Banana Blueberry Smoothie
Serves 2
1 cup nonfat plain yogurt
1/2 cup blueberries
2 ripe bananas

Peel the bananas, slice them in half, and place on a tray. Put into the freezer and freeze until they are solid. Put the frozen bananas into a blender, add the blueberries and yogurt, and blend until smooth.

BARLEY

Barley is a member of the grass family and is mainly a cereal grain. It has a long history: The cultivated barley we have today was once a wild grass that most experts believe originated in the Near East, although some argue it was China or Ethiopia. Barley was first cultivated around 10,000 B.C. in western Asia, and the ancient peoples made barley bread long before they domesticated wheat. Travelers brought barley to Spain in the fifth century B.C. before they carried it to France and Germany. The people of Turkey, Syria, Egypt, and Greece are responsible for developing the art of making beer from barley. Drinking beer, however, is not the preferred way to get your barley.

The first barley crop grown in North America was in

Massachusetts in 1620. Today barley is the world's fourth most important crop and it is a staple in many countries. The United States is the third largest producer of barley, yet most of it is used for animal feed and to make beer. Its dietary nutritional value is largely unappreciated.

Barley is available in several forms, each of which differs somewhat in nutritional value and in how it can be used.

- **Hulled:** This is the most nutritious form because the bran is still intact. It is usually only available in health food stores but worth the trip. It is brownish in color and has a nutty flavor.

- **Pearled:** This is the most common form and the easiest to find in supermarkets. It has undergone a polishing process that removes the hull and bran layers, leaving it a pearly white in color.

- **Scotch barley:** Also known as pot barley, it is less refined than pearled barley and has part of its hull. It is not always easy to find in stores.

- **Barley grits:** The grain is cracked, toasted, or parboiled, then dried, which makes it into a fast-cooking product.

- **Barley flakes or rolled barley:** These forms look like rolled oats and can be found in cereals.

- **Barley flour:** The flour is finely ground and has a delicate sweetness. Because it has a very low

gluten content, it can be blended with other flours
for baking.

NUTRITIONAL VALUE—HULLED BARLEY
$1/2$ cup cooked
Calories: 326
Fiber: 16 g, 50%
Iron: 3.3 mg, 41% DRI
Potassium: 416 mg, 9% DRI
Selenium: 34 mg, 62% DRI
Zinc: 2.5 mg, 23% DRI

NUTRITIONAL VALUE—PEARLED BARLEY
$1/2$ cup cooked
Calories: 97
Fiber: 3 g, 9%
Iron: 1 mg, 12% DRI

Why Barley Is Heart-Healthy
If you want to get the most out of your barley, you need
to turn to the hulled form. Ounce for ounce, this whole-
grain variety has more fiber and more of nearly every
mineral that both hulled and pearled types share. Therefore, although barley overall is a heart-healthy food, you
get the most bang for your buck if you choose the hulled
form.

• Barley is an excellent source of beta-glucans,
  which have the ability to reduce serum cholesterol, and especially low-density lipoprotein (LDL,
  the "bad") cholesterol. Beta-glucans are part of
  the fiber found in the cell walls of barley. Some
  varieties of barley (especially hulled) contain up

to three times the level of beta-glucans as most varieties of oats.

- Barley is a good source of the mineral selenium, which has been shown to be important in patients who have coronary artery disease (CAD). A recent study (2008) published in the *American Heart Journal* reported that selenium supplementation improves the activity of the potent antioxidant glutathione peroxidase-1, which is beneficial for people who have CAD.

- The Food and Drug Administration has recognized that barley is a reliable source of betaglucan soluble fiber, which means barley products can include labeling with a health claim stating that it can help reduce the risk of coronary heart disease.

- Potassium is necessary to properly transmit electrical signals in the heart. People who take diuretics often have low levels of potassium, a condition that can disrupt the normal electrical impulses and result in irregular heartbeats. Barley provides a very good amount of potassium.

RECIPE

It is recommended that you presoak barley the night before you plan to cook and use it. The ratio of barley to water is 1 cup of barley and 3 cups of water. Soak overnight or at least five to six hours. To cook presoaked barley, bring the barley and water to a boil in an uncovered pot. Once it is boiling, reduce the heat and cover. Allow the barley to simmer for 45 minutes. (For non-presoaked barley, cook for 1½ to 2 hours.) Do not add salt to the barley until after it is cooked. A sign that barley is done: about 20 percent of the barley grains will have burst open.

Rainbow Barley Salad
Serves 8
1 cup hulled barley
3 cups water
1 can black or kidney beans, drained
2/3 cup finely chopped red onion
1/2 cup chopped red bell pepper
1/2 cup chopped green bell pepper
1 cup strawberries, cut into small pieces
4 Tbs chopped fresh cilantro
2/3 cup white wine vinegar
1/3 cup olive oil
1 tsp ground black pepper
1 tsp chili powder
1 tsp dry mustard
1/2 tsp salt
1 tsp honey

In saucepan, bring the water to a boil and add the barley. Cook until tender. In a large bowl, combine the cooked barley, beans, strawberries, onion, bell pepper, and cilantro. In a small saucepan, combine the vinegar, olive oil, honey, salt, pepper, chili powder, and dry mustard. Heat until it bubbles. Pour the dressing over the barley-vegetable mixture. Refrigerate, covered, for at least 4 hours.

BEANS

Dried beans have been a staple of the diet of many peoples around the world for thousands of years. The birthplaces of beans, so to speak, are Africa, Asia, and the Middle East. Besides the fact that they are loaded with protein and other essential nutrients, beans have a long shelf life, which means you can store them, uncooked, for several years. In the days before refrigeration, that benefit meant the difference between life and death when other food was scarce! Apparently the Egyptians took the storage benefit one step further: beans that were placed in the tombs of ancient pharaohs have been found to be viable even to this day.

Beans are an annual crop, and most varieties are planted in the spring and harvested in the fall. From white beans to black, kidneys to Great Northern, pink to red, beans can be prepared in scores of ways, they provide many health benefits, and they are economical.

NUTRITIONAL VALUE—PINTO BEANS
1/2 cup cooked
Calories: 122
Fiber: 7.8 g, 24%
Iron: 1.8 mg, 22% DRI
Potassium: 375 mg, 8% DRI
Folic acid: 148 mcg, 37% DRI

NUTRITIONAL VALUE—KIDNEY BEANS
1/2 cup cooked
Calories: 112
Fiber: 5.7 g, 18%
Iron: 2 mg, 25% DRI

Potassium: 358 mg, 7% DRI
Folic acid: 115 mcg, 29% DRI

Why Beans Are Heart-Healthy

According to a study published in the *Journal of the American College of Nutrition,* "Including dry beans in a health-promoting diet is especially important in meeting the major dietary recommendations to reduce risk for chronic diseases such as coronary heart disease, diabetes mellitus, obesity and cancer." That's a very good endorsement for what many people today consider to be the poor man's protein.

But wise is the man/woman/child, and healthy too, who includes beans in their diet. Beans are a great source of complex carbohydrates, soluble fiber, iron, and folic acid, yet they contain little or no fat and have no cholesterol. Blackeyed peas are especially high in folic acid, which helps fight heart disease. Studies show that beans can help lower cholesterol levels, balance blood sugar levels, and assist with weight loss.

RECIPE

This recipe combines several heart-healthy foods. You can use canned beans, but we suggest you buy salt-free varieties or rinse salted ones.

Bean and Kale Salad
Serves 4–6
4 cups chopped kale
1/2 medium onion, diced
1/2 fennel bulb, diced
1/2 cup garbanzo beans, cooked and drained

1/2 cup black beans, cooked and drained
1/2 cup pinto beans, cooked and drained
1/2 cup celery, chopped
4 cloves garlic, minced

Dressing
2 Tbs balsamic vinegar
2 Tbs white vinegar
1/4 cup water
1/4 cup olive oil
1 tsp dried dill
1 tsp fennel seeds

Combine all the beans and vegetables in a large bowl. In a separate bowl, whisk the dressing ingredients. Pour the dressing over the vegetables, mix well, and chill until ready to eat.

BELL PEPPERS

Bell peppers, be they red, green, yellow, purple, orange, or black, originated in South America from wild seeds that likely date back to 5000 B.C. Because pepper plants adapt well to both tropical and temperate climates, they easily took hold throughout the world as the Portuguese and Spanish explorers carried the seeds with them as they traveled. Today bell peppers are grown around the world, but the main producers are China, Turkey, Spain, Romania, Nigeria, and Mexico.

Just a few fun facts about bell peppers: All bell peppers have a recessive gene that eliminates capsaicin, the substance that makes other peppers hot. Red bell peppers are the sole source of pimiento and paprika, which are important ingredients in Creole, Mexican, and Portuguese dishes.

NUTRITIONAL VALUE—GREEN BELL PEPPER
1 cup chopped
Calories: 30
Fiber: 2.5 g, 8%
Folic acid: 15 mcg, 4% DRI
Potassium: 261 mg, 6% DRI
Vitamin A: 551 IU, 18% DRI
Vitamin B_6: 0.3 mg, 18% DRI
Vitamin C: 120 mg, 133% DRI
Vitamin K: 11 mcg

NUTRITIONAL VALUE—RED BELL PEPPER
1 cup chopped
Calories: 46
Fiber: 3.1 g, 10%
Calcium: 10 mg
Folic acid: 69 mcg, 17% DRI
Potassium: 314 mg, 7% DRI
Vitamin A: 4,665 IU, 156% DRI
Vitamin B_6: 0.4 mg, 24% DRI
Vitamin C: 190 mg, 211% DRI
Vitamin K: 7.3 mg

NUTRITIONAL VALUE—YELLOW BELL PEPPER
1 cup chopped
Calories: 42
Fiber: 1.4 g, 4%
Calcium: 17 mg
Folic acid: 41 mcg, 10% DRI

Potassium: 331 mg, 7% DRI
Vitamin A: 312 IU, 10% DRI
Vitamin B_6: 0.26 mg, 15% DRI
Vitamin C: 286 mg, 317% DRI

Why Bell Peppers Are Heart-Healthy

Regardless of their color, bell peppers are a rich source of vitamins, minerals, and phytonutrients. The level of each nutrient varies among the different colors of bells, but overall they are a hearty bunch. Here's what we mean.

- Bell peppers provide a good amount of folic acid and vitamin B_6, both of which are needed to help reduce high levels of the heart-damaging amino acid called homocysteine.

- The fiber in bell peppers can help lower cholesterol levels.

- Bell peppers contain a good source of vitamin K, which promotes normal blood clotting.

- Red bell peppers are a good source of lycopene. A study published in the *American Journal of Clinical Nutrition* (2004) reported that dietary lycopene may significantly reduce the risk of heart disease. Researchers found that women who had the highest levels of the antioxidant in their blood had a 34 percent reduced risk of the disease compared with women who had lower levels of the nutrient.

• The antioxidants vitamins A and C help prevent free radical damage to the heart. They also prevent the accumulation of plaque on the walls of the arteries, which can block blood flow and cause heart attack and stroke.

RECIPE
This recipe calls for four different colors of peppers. If you can get more, go for it!

Four Pepper Salad
Serves 6–8
1 each: red, green, yellow, and orange bell pepper,
cored and seeded
1 small purple onion, peeled
1 small carrot, grated
1/4 cup chopped fresh basil
2 Tbs rice vinegar
1 Tbs sesame oil
Salt and black pepper to taste
2 Tbs chopped almonds or walnuts

Slice the peppers and onion into matchstick-size pieces and put in a large bowl. Add the carrots and basil and sprinkle with salt and pepper. Add the rice vinegar and sesame oil, stir to mix and chill, covered, for at least one hour before serving. Before serving, toss again and sprinkle on the nuts.

BERRIES
Blueberries, blackberries, lingonberries, bilberries, cranberries, raspberries, strawberries—they're colorful, deli-

cious, healthful, and a huge favorite among people of all ages. Most berries can trace their origins from the Americas. The modern strawberry, for example, is the result of cross-breeding of two New World varieties— one originally found in Virginia and the other from the west coast of South America.

The Native Americans introduced blueberries to the colonists, who quickly decided they loved the small berries both raw and dried. While the wild varieties are small, a type called highbush, first cultivated in the 1920s by Dr. F.V. Coville, are up to four times larger than their wild cousins. Blackberries claim more than 2,000 varieties, and raspberries have a history as a medicinal fruit that healed wounds.

NUTRITIONAL VALUE—BLUEBERRIES
1 cup fresh
Calories: 84
Fiber: 3.6 g, 11%
Vitamin C: 14 mg, 16% DRI

NUTRITIONAL VALUE—STRAWBERRIES
1 cup fresh
Calories: 53
Fiber: 3.3 g, 10%
Folic acid: 40 mcg, 10% DRI
Vitamin C: 98 mg, 109% DRI

NUTRITIONAL VALUE—RASPBERRIES
1 cup fresh
Calories: 64
Fiber: 8 g, 25%
Manganese: 0.8 mg, 35% DRI
Vitamin C: 32 mg, 36% DRI

Why Berries Are Heart-Healthy

Berries are a powerhouse of antioxidants, polyphenols, and other nutrients that offer advantages for the heart. Take the blueberry. When scientists put this little blue orb through the paces, they discovered that it has one of the highest antioxidant potency values of any food. Let's look at some berry research.

- In several studies of blueberries, experts found that the antioxidants they contained helped prevent oxidative and inflammatory stress on the lining of red blood cells and the blood vessels, two critical factors in preventing heart disease. Overall, in fact, the antioxidants in berries inhibit the oxidation of low-density lipoproteins (LDLs), which can help prevent the formation of plaque in the arteries and reduce the incidence of heart attack.

- In 2008, a double-blind, placebo-controlled study published in the *American Journal of Clinical Nutrition* reported on the ability of several different berries to reduce blood pressure and also raise the level of "good" cholesterol, high-density lipoprotein (HDL). The study used a combination of bilberries, strawberries, black currants, and lingonberries because they wanted to maximize the intake of polyphenols. The study's authors reported that polyphenols and vitamin C were "the most likely berry constituents to exert effects." They believe their findings help explain why a diet rich in fruits and vegetables protects against cardiovascular disease.

RECIPE

Just because this recipe is a sundae doesn't mean it's only for dessert. Treat yourself and your heart to this berry treat for breakfast sometimes.

Berry Berry Sundae
1/2 cup strawberries
1/2 cup raspberries
1/2 cup blueberries
1/2 tsp lemon juice
2 cups nonfat vanilla frozen yogurt

Reserve a few of each of the berries, then puree the remaining berries with the lemon juice in a blender. Serve over frozen yogurt and top with the remaining berries.

BROCCOLI

Did you know that broccoli florets are really flowers? Although they may not look like the flowers you are used to seeing, a broccoli bouquet would certainly bring a smile—and a look of surprise—to anyone's face while also delivering a healthy dose of nutrition.

Broccoli, known in the scientific world as *Brassica oleracea italica,* originated in the Mediterranean. The ancient Etruscans developed broccoli from a cabbage. Broccoli has been cultivated since the 1500s, but it did not become popular in the United States until the early 1920s. The color of broccoli varieties range from deep sage to dark green and purplish-green. One of the most popular types of broccoli consumed in the United States is Calabrese (named after the Italian province Calabria where it was first grown), or Italian green.

NUTRITIONAL VALUE—BROCCOLI
½ cup chopped, cooked
Calories: 27
Fiber: 2.6 g, 8%
Vitamin A: 1207 IU, 40% DRI
Vitamin C: 50 mg, 56% DRI
Folic acid: 84 mcg, 21% DRI

Why Broccoli Is Heart-Healthy
A little broccoli goes a long way when it comes to nutrition. Ounce for ounce, boiled broccoli has more vitamin C than an orange, and just one medium spear has three times more fiber than a slice of wheat bran bread.

- University of Connecticut researchers found some heartening news about broccoli. For one month they fed broccoli extract to a group of rats while another group received water rather than the extract. The scientists then performed various tests on the rats, and those that had eaten the broccoli extract had less heart damage when they were oxygen deprived, better ability to pump blood, and higher levels of important heart chemicals during oxygen deprivation.

- Broccoli also has a positive effect on cholesterol because it is an excellent source of indole-3-carbinol, which can significantly reduce the secretion of apolipoprotein B-100 (ApoB), the main apolipoprotein of LDL cholesterol and the substance that transports cholesterol to tissues. ApoB also is associated with the formation of plaque in the blood vessels.

- The kaempferol in broccoli is heart friendly, according to a study in women, which found that the phytonutrient reduced the risk of coronary heart disease.

- The antioxidants beta-carotene and vitamin C in broccoli may help reduce the risk of heart disease.

RECIPE

This recipe combines three heart-healthy ingredients in one easy, delicious treat.

Broccoli and Sweet Potato
Serves 2
2 small sweet potatoes, about 12 ounces
2 cups broccoli florets
1/2 cup kidney beans
1/4 tsp curry powder
1/8 tsp garlic powder
1 tsp olive oil
Black pepper to taste

Scrub the potatoes and cut into small cubes. Cut the broccoli into bite-size pieces. Steam the potatoes and broccoli until tender. In a bowl combine the beans, curry, garlic powder, and olive oil. Add the potatoes and broccoli, mix well, and serve warm or chilled.

BROWN RICE

Rice is a grain that is a member of the grass family. Its exact origins are not certain, but many experts believe rice was first discovered in the wilds of India around 3000 B.C. It is consumed by about half the world's population and is one of the few foods in the world that is completely nonallergenic and gluten-free.

Rice is naturally brown; it is covered with a hull and several bran layers of kernel which are removed during the processing of white rice. Brown rice is more nutritious than white rice because the bran contains a concentration of nutrients and fiber that are eliminated during processing. In fact, the milling and polishing that transforms brown rice into white rice removes about 33 percent of its iron and vitamin B_3, 50 percent of its phosphorus and manganese, 80 percent of vitamin B_1, ninety percent of vitamin B_6, and all of the fiber. Other nutrients are also reduced or removed.

NUTRITIONAL VALUE—BROWN RICE
1 cup cooked
Calories: 216
Fiber: 3.5 g, 11%
Manganese: 2.1 mg, 91% DRI
Niacin: 3 mg, 19% DRI
Selenium: 19 mcg, 36% DRI
Thiamin: 0.19 mg, 16% DRI
Zinc: 1.2 mg, 11% DRI

Why Brown Rice Is Heart-Healthy
Brown rice is cholesterol-free, virtually fat-free, and contains five times more vitamin E and three times more magnesium than white rice. These and other nutrients make brown rice good for your heart.

- The selenium in brown rice is a potent antioxidant that helps prevent heart disease.

- The ability of brown rice to help reduce cholesterol comes from several factors, one of which is fiber. A meta-analysis of seven studies that looked at whole grains, including brown rice, found that people whose diets had the highest dietary fiber intake had a 29 percent lower risk of cardiovascular disease compared with people who had the lowest fiber intake. Fiber also helps keep blood sugar levels under control, high levels of which are a risk factor for heart disease.

- Brown rice contains an oil-rich germ that lowers cholesterol levels. In a study published in the *American Journal of Clinical Nutrition,* researchers assessed the impact of a diet that included defatted rice bran with one that contained regular rice bran oil. Participants who consumed rice bran oil in their diet had their LDL (low-density lipoprotein) cholesterol levels reduced by 7 percent while subjects who ate the defatted rice bran did not see a reduction.

- Brown rice contains polyunsaturated fatty acids, plant sterols, and saponins, which have cholesterol-lowering effects.

- Magnesium is important for heart health because it prevents calcium from activating nerves, which in turn keeps blood vessels relaxed. An insufficient amount of magnesium can contribute to high blood pressure and spasms of the heart muscle.

- Brown rice contains phytoestrogens, which may have an effect on blood cholesterol and elasticity of blood vessels.

- Research indicates that regular consumption of whole grains like brown rice reduces the risk of type 2 diabetes, which is a major risk factor for heart disease.

- Brown rice is a rich source of lignans, which are converted in the body to enterolactone and enterodiole. Studies show that blood levels of enterolactone help reduce the risk of cardiovascular-related death.

RECIPE
Here's a recipe that brings together several heart-healthy foods to maximize the benefits.

Brown Rice and Asparagus
Serves 4–6
1 cup red beans, cooked (you can use unsalted canned beans)
1/2 cup celery, chopped
1 bunch asparagus, cut into 1-inch pieces
1 medium onion, chopped
2 cloves garlic, minced
3 cups cooked brown rice
1/2 cup almond slivers
3 Tbs olive oil
Salt to taste

Dressing
1 clove garlic, chopped fine
1 tsp dried dill
1/4 cup tahini
1/8 cup lemon juice
2 Tbs olive oil
2 Tbs hot water
1/2 tsp sea salt

To prepare the dressing, whisk together the garlic, tahini, lemon juice, and olive oil. Add the hot water to thin it and then add the salt. Set aside.

In a large skillet, heat the oil over medium high heat. Add the beans, garlic, and onions and stir for about two minutes. Add the asparagus, salt, and cover the skillet with a lid for 1 to 2 minutes until the asparagus begins to get soft. Stir in the rice and almonds and add more salt if desired. Place the mixture in a large bowl and drizzle with the dressing, reserving some of the dressing for individual taste preferences.

BULGAR

Bulgar, also known as bulgar wheat, bulgur, and bulghur, is a Middle Eastern way to prepare wheat so that it keeps nearly all of the germ and bran. It originated in the Mediterranean area and to this day is a main staple of the Middle Eastern diet. Its importance as a food source was recognized by the Chinese as far back as 2800 B.C., when Chinese emperor Shen Nung called it one of the five sacred crops, joining rice, soybeans, millet, and barley. The ability of bulgar to resist mold and attack by pests and its long shelf life made it a critical food item for primitive and ancient peoples.

The ancient way to prepare bulgar was to boil the wheat in large pots until it was completely cooked, and then spread it out on flat roofs to dry. This process is still used today by some villagers, and the basic concept is still followed despite modern processing techniques.

NUTRITIONAL VALUE—BULGAR
1 cup, cooked
Calories: 151
Fiber: 8.0 g, 25%
Iron: 1.7 mg, 21% DRI
Niacin: 1.8 mg, 11% DRI
Magnesium: 58 mg, 14% DRI
Manganese: 1.1 mg, 48% DRI

Why Bulgar Is Heart-Healthy

In a word, "fiber" is the main reason bulgar is heart-friendly. One serving of bulgar provides about one third of the daily requirement of fiber. It is also a good source of iron, niacin, and magnesium, and an excellent source of manganese. Why is any of this important for the heart?

- Fiber is critical for preventing heart disease. In an exceptionally large review published in the *Archives of Internal Medicine*, experts analyzed the data from 10 studies that included 91,058 men and 245,186 women and estimated the association between dietary fiber intake and the risk of coronary heart disease. They found that each 10-gram per day intake of dietary fiber was associated with a 14 percent decreased risk of all coronary events and a 27 percent decreased risk of coronary death.

• Bulgar is an excellent source of manganese. This often-ignored mineral plays an important role in heart health, in that a deficiency of manganese is associated with high cholesterol, high blood pressure, and heart disorders. Manganese also enhances the absorption of magnesium, another mineral that plays a significant role in heart health. Coincidentally, bulgar also contains a good amount of magnesium!

• If you want to reduce your intake of animal protein and saturated fat, which is recommended as part of a heart-healthy diet, then bulgar is a good non-animal source of protein. One cup of cooked bulgar provides six grams of protein, and so it is a good alternative for red meat.

RECIPE

Bulgar can be used in recipes that call for rice or cous cous, and it has more nutritional value than these grains. One of the most popular dishes that uses bulgar is tabouli, so we've offered you one version below.

Tabouli
Serves 6–8
1 cup bulgar wheat, dry
1½ cups boiling water

¹/₄ cup lemon juice
¹/₄ cup olive oil
1 tsp salt (optional)
2 cloves garlic, minced
4 scallions, minced
1 cup of minced parsley
10 mint leaves or 2 Tbs dried mint
2 medium tomatoes, diced

Place the bulgar in a bowl, cover it with the boiling water, and let it stand for at least 20 minutes. Add the lemon juice, garlic, oil, salt, and pepper and mix well. Cover and refrigerate for one hour. Thirty minutes before you plan to serve the tabouli, combine the bulgar and the flavorings and mix well. Refrigerate.

CARROTS

Thousands of years ago, when carrots first popped onto the scene in central Asia and the Middle East, they were deep purple to lavender in color, which reflected the phytonutrient pigment called anthocyanin. The familiar orange version we see today originated as a yellow variety in Afghanistan.

Carrots became popular in Europe during the Renaissance, but it was not until the beginning of the seventeenth century that agriculturists in Europe cultivated different varieties. One of the results was an orange carrot that had a better texture than its predecessors, and it became favored over the purple varieties. Soon after that, carrots were introduced into North America. Today, the world's largest carrot producers are the United States, France, England, Poland, China, and Japan. Carrots are available in yellow, orange, black, white, red, and purple varieties.

NUTRITIONAL VALUE—CARROTS
½ cup cooked
Calories: 27
Fiber: 2.3 g, 7%
Vitamin A: 13,288 IU, 429% DRI

Why Carrots Are Heart-Healthy

Carrots get an A+, and that grade is for its very high level of vitamin A/beta-carotene and other carotenoids, including lutein, lycopene, and zeaxanthin. What is so special about carrots that they deserve this excellent grade?

- Several epidemiological studies have examined the relationship between a diet high in carotenoids and heart disease and they found that high-carotenoid diets are associated with a reduced risk of heart disease. In one study of 1,300 elderly adults, those who consumed at least one serving of carrots and/or squash (also high in carotenoids) daily had a 60 percent reduced risk of heart attacks compared with their peers who ate less than one serving of such foods daily.

- Several studies indicate that carrot consumption can effectively lower cholesterol levels. One theory is that this reduction may be related to a type of fiber called calcium pectate, which is found in carrots.

RECIPE

Raw carrots are one of the easiest and more popular snacks, whether they are eaten alone or with a dip. Cooked carrots have found their way into a wide variety of recipes, from appetizers to desserts. Here's a medley you can enjoy alone or as a side dish.

Carrots with Kick
Serves 2–4
2 large carrots, cut into wedges
12 black olives
6 radishes, sliced thin
1 clove garlic, chopped
1/4 tsp paprika
1/2 tsp ground cumin
1 pinch cayenne pepper
1 pinch cinnamon
Juice of one fresh lemon
1/8 cup olive oil

Boil or steam the carrots until they are tender. Rinse them under cold water, then place them in a shallow pan with the radishes and olives. Mix the remaining ingredients together to create a marinade. Pour the marinade over the vegetables and allow to sit for about 1 hour.

DARK CHOCOLATE

Is it true that chocolate is good for the heart? Well, that news just makes the heart beat faster for lots of chocoholics. But before you run down to the store and stock up on your favorite chocolate bars, we need to clarify the opening statement: *dark* chocolate is good for the heart, and only in moderation.

People have had a love affair with chocolate for millennia. The secret of the cacao tree and its pods was discovered about 2,000 years ago by the natives of Central America and Mexico. The ancient Aztecs and Mayans were the first to mix ground cacao seeds with seasonings to make a beverage. When the Spanish conquistadors visited the Americas, they brought the cacao seeds back to Spain, and it wasn't long before chocolate drinks gained popularity all across Europe.

Chocolate made the transition from its liquid (beverage)—and quite expensive—form to a solid form when the Industrial Revolution took hold in the late eighteenth to early nineteenth century. Once solid chocolate was possible, new machinery was able to mass-produce it, and the cost was dramatically reduced. That's when chocolate became available to the masses.

NUTRITIONAL VALUE—DARK CHOCOLATE
1 ounce
Calories: 155
Fiber: 2 g, 6%
Iron: 2.3 mg, 28% DRI
Potassium: 161 mg, 3% DRI

Why Dark Chocolate Is Heart-Healthy

If you read the ingredient label on a bar of dark chocolate, you won't see anything that indicates it is a heart-healthy food. That's because dark chocolate—but not milk or white chocolate—contains high levels of plant phenols that act as antioxidants. Eating 2 ounces (50 grams) of plain dark chocolate a day with a minimum content of 70 percent chocolate solids can be good for your health. Although dark chocolate has benefits not found in other types of chocolate, it still has lots of fat and calories, so the temptation to eat a lot of this sweet needs to be reined in. Here's what the studies say.

- A study published in the *Journal of the American Medical Association* in 2003 found that dark chocolate lowers high blood pressure. The participants in the study ate a 100-gram dark chocolate or milk chocolate candy bar daily for 14 days (and skipped other foods to make up for the 480 calories in the candy). At the end of the study, those who ate the dark chocolate had a significant decline in blood pressure while those who ate the milk chocolate did not.

- The antioxidants in dark chocolate destroy free radicals that are implicated in heart disease. Do not drink milk with your chocolate, because it may interfere with the body's ability to absorb the antioxidants and thus negate the benefits from the chocolate. In a study from Italy's National Institute for Food and Nutrition Research, the investigators tried three approaches: Twelve men and women ate either 100 grams of dark chocolate by itself, 100 grams of dark chocolate with a small glass of whole milk, or 200 grams of milk chocolate. The participants who ate the dark chocolate alone had the most total antioxidants in their blood.

- Dark chocolate also contains high levels of epicatechin, a flavonoid. Flavonoids prevent accumulation of plaque in the blood vessels, reduce the risk of blood clots, and slow down the mechanisms that can result in clogged arteries. A study investigated the impact of epicatechin on the heart. Two groups of healthy adults ate a dark chocolate candy bar daily for two weeks: one group got a bar that contained epicatechin, the other group ate epicatechin-free chocolate. The researchers then evaluated how well the blood vessels dilated and relaxed in all of the participants, which is an indication of healthy blood vessel function. The subjects who ate the epicatechin-laced dark chocolate had blood vessels that performed significantly better than those in the other group.

RECIPE

This recipe is a little decadent, but everyone deserves some sweetness in their life. Its saving grace? It combines two heart-healthy foods.

Chocolate Dipped Strawberries
6 oz dark chocolate
3 Tbs half and half cream
1/2 Tbs unsalted butter
20 large or 30 medium strawberries

In a one-quart glass bowl combine the chocolate and cream. Heat in a microwave on high about 1 to 2 minutes, stirring several times, until smooth. Add butter and

*stir until it melts. Dip each strawberry into the chocolate
mixture and allow the excess chocolate to drip back into
the bowl. Line a baking sheet with waxed paper or foil
and transfer the coated berries to the sheet. Refrigerate
the coated berries until the chocolate is set, about 20 to
30 minutes.*

EGGPLANT

Eggplant is a uniquely shaped vegetable that belongs to
the nightshade family, which also includes tomatoes, potatoes, and bell peppers. Although eggplant comes in several varieties, the most popular has deep purple skin with
a glossy finish and a cream-colored, spongy flesh. Other
varieties include those with lavender, orange, jade green,
and yellow-white skin. Eggplant varieties range in size
from that of a small peach to a large zucchini. Regardless
of the variety, eggplant generally has a slightly bitter taste.

Eggplant originated in India, where it grew wild, and it
was first cultivated in China in the fifth century B.C. The
odd-shaped vegetable was introduced to Africa before the
Middle Ages and found its way to Italy in the fourteenth
century, after which it spread throughout Europe and the
Middle East. Explorers from Europe eventually brought it
to the New World.

Because the earlier varieties of eggplant had a strong
bitter taste, early Europeans believed that it could cause
insanity, leprosy, and cancer. Thus it was not until some
innovative individuals developed new, better-tasting varieties of eggplant that the vegetable gained a positive repu-
tation and an honored place in the cuisines of European
countries. Today, the leading producers of eggplant are
Italy, Turkey, Egypt, China, and Japan.

NUTRITIONAL VALUE—EGGPLANT, BOILED
One cup, cubes
Calories: 33
Fiber: 2.5 g, 8%

Why Eggplant Is Heart-Healthy
The nutritional value table on eggplant does not look impressive, but what you can't see is that the vegetable is a rich source of phenolic compounds, which were discovered by researchers at the U.S. Agricultural Service. The main phenolic compound in eggplant is chlorogenic acid, which is one of the most potent free-radical fighters found in plants. Among its many benefits is its ability to battle cholesterol. Some of the virtues of eggplant can be seen below.

- In several studies, eggplant was given to laboratory animals, and blood cholesterol levels were significantly reduced. Eggplant also caused the blood vessels to relax and improved blood flow. Experts credit several phytonutrients with these benefits, including nasunin.

- Nasunin also acts as a chelator of iron, which means it attaches itself to iron and helps eliminate it from the body. Although iron is necessary for good health, too much iron is associated with an increased risk of heart disease. Postmenopausal women and men are more likely to have excess iron. By chelating iron, nasunin reduces the risk of heart problems and protects against the formation of free radicals, which can damage the heart.

RECIPE

If you are expecting an eggplant parmesan recipe, we're sorry to disappoint you. But we believe this eggplant stew will become one of your favorites, perfect for lunch or dinner.

Eggplant Stew
Serves 3–4
1/2 cup chopped onion
1/4 cup chopped carrots
1/4 cup chopped celery
1 large eggplant, peeled and cubed
1 bell pepper, diced
2 cloves garlic, minced
2 1/2 cups vegetable broth, low-salt
8 oz red or white beans
1 cup chopped spinach
1 can diced tomatoes with liquid
1 tsp salt
2 Tbs chopped cilantro
1/4 tsp cayenne

Saute the onions, carrots, celery, eggplant, bell pepper, and garlic in a large skillet with spray-on oil until lightly brown. Add the broth, beans, tomatoes, spinach, and seasonings. Simmer for 30 minutes or until vegetables are tender.

FIGS

Whether they are dried or fresh, figs have been a favorite food for millennia. Figs were mentioned in ancient writings and in the Bible, and are believed to have been first cultivated in Egypt. These sweet fruits were carried to ancient Crete and then made their way to Greece around the ninth century BC. When the Greeks familiarized themselves with figs, they so honored them that they did not allow any high-quality fruits to be exported. The ancient Romans considered the fig to be sacred because the founders of Rome, Romulus and Remus, rested under a fig tree.

Spanish explorers brought figs to the Western hemisphere, and by the late nineteenth century Spanish missionaries planted fig trees in San Diego, California. Today California is one of the primary producers of figs, along with Greece, Turkey, Spain, and Portugal. California figs are usually available from June through September, while some European varieties are available through the fall.

Figs grow on the ficus tree *(Ficus carica)*, and can vary significantly in color, depending on the variety. Most figs are dried, which allows them to be enjoyed year round.

NUTRITIONAL VALUE—FIGS, RAW
One large (2½")
Calories: 47
Fiber: 1.9 mg, 6%
Calcium: 22 mg
Potassium: 148 mg, 3% DRI

NUTRITIONAL VALUE—FIGS, DRIED
½ cup
Calories: 185
Fiber: 7.3 mg, 23%
Calcium: 120 mg
Iron: 1.5 mg, 19% DRI
Magnesium: 50 mg, 12% DRI
Potassium: 506 mg, 11% DRI

Why Figs Are Heart-Healthy

Although fresh, raw figs are a tasty treat, their nutritional value pales when compared with dried figs. But don't stop at the fruit itself: Even fig leaves have some heart-friendly benefits. Animal study results show that fig leaves can reduce triglyceride levels. For now, however, it's best to focus on the fruit and not the leaves.

- The high potassium and very low sodium levels in figs can help to control blood pressure. In the Dietary Approaches to Stop Hypertension (DASH) study, participants who ate fruits and vegetables (which provided more potassium, magnesium, and calcium) instead of snacks and sugary foods had reduced their blood pressure by an average of 5.5 points (systolic) over 3.0 points (diastolic) after eight weeks compared with people who ate the standard American diet. Note that dried figs are especially good sources of potassium, magnesium, and calcium.

- The high fiber content in dried figs contributes to the elimination of cholesterol from the body and thus reduces the risk of heart disease and stroke.

- Figs are also a good source of the mineral manganese, which, when not available in sufficient amounts, is associated with an increased risk of heart disease.

RECIPE

This recipe combines several heart-friendly foods in a fruity salsa that can be served with fish, tofu, chicken, or turkey, or spread on a bagel.

Figgy Fruity Salsa
Makes 3 cups
1¹/₂ cups diced red bell pepper
1 cup diced figs
¹/₂ cup diced fresh mango
¹/₂ cup diced red onion
¹/₂ cup diced apple
¹/₄ cup chopped cilantro
¹/₂ jalapeno chili pepper, seeded and minced
3 Tbs lime juice
1 tsp minced garlic
¹/₂ tsp salt
¹/₂ cup chopped almonds or walnuts

Combine all ingredients except the nuts in a bowl. Cover and chill for one hour. Stir in the nuts just before you serve it.

FLAXSEED

Flaxseed comes from the flax plant, which has its origins in the Stone Age. The seeds are slightly larger than sesame seeds and their shells are hard, shiny, and smooth. Flax is either brown or golden and the seeds range from reddish brown to deep amber.

The ancient Greeks used flaxseed for food, and both they and the ancient Romans revered it for medicinal purposes. Flax lost its popularity after these great civilizations declined, but it was revived by the emperor Charlemagne, who praised its value as a food, medicine, and fiber for making linen. He was so enamored with flaxseed that he made its cultivation and consumption mandatory.

The early colonists in North America brought flax with them, and it was first planted in Canada. Today Canada is the world's largest producer of flax and flaxseed.

NUTRITIONAL VALUE—FLAXSEED
2 tablespoons whole seeds
Calories: 95
Fiber: 5.4 g, 17%
Magnesium: 70 mg, 17% DRI
Manganese: 0.64 mg, 28% DRI
Folic acid: 54 mcg, 14% DRI

Why Flaxseed Is Heart-Healthy
Seeds are one of nature's nutritional wonders, as they typically pack a lot of power into something very small. Flaxseed is a good source of magnesium, manganese, and fiber, but its real heart benefits are in the omega-3 fatty acids. Here's a rundown of the benefits of flaxseed.

- Omega-3 fatty acids are an important ingredient in the production of substances that reduce the formation of blood clots. This activity is critical to reduce the risk of stroke and heart attack in people who have atherosclerosis or heart disease.

- Omega-3 fatty acids have a positive impact on blood pressure. The INTERMAP study (International Study of Macro- and Micro-nutrients and

Blood Pressure) studied the dietary habits of 4,680 adults to determine their intake of omega-3 fatty acids from fish, nuts, seeds, and vegetable oils. Participants who consumed more omega-3 fatty acids as a percentage of their daily calorie intake had a lower blood pressure reading than those who consumed less of the fatty acids.

- Eating foods high in fiber, such as flaxseed, reduces the risk of coronary heart disease and cardiovascular disease. A study of nearly 10,000 adults followed for 19 years found that those who ate the most fiber daily (21 grams) had 12 percent less coronary heart disease and 11 percent less cardiovascular disease compared with those who ate the least amount (5 grams daily).

- The magnesium in flaxseed can help reduce high blood pressure and thus the risk of heart attack and stroke.

RECIPE

You can grind flaxseeds in a seed or coffee grinder. This improves their digestibility and nutritional value.

Just the Flax Salsa
Makes 2 cups
2 cups diced fresh tomato
1/2 cup fresh or frozen kernel corn
3 Tbs diced onion
1 jalapeno pepper, minced
1 clove garlic, minced
2 Tbs lime juice

3 Tbs ground flaxseed
2 Tbs chopped cilantro
2 tsp whole flaxseed, ground

In a bowl, combine all the ingredients except the flaxseed and cilantro. Cover and refrigerate for 2 hours. Before serving, stir in the flaxseed and cilantro.

GREENS

Some people jokingly refer to leafy green vegetables as rabbit food, but the joke is on you if you shun these hearty-healthy foods. Greens is a term that includes a long list of leafy vegetables, encompassing but not limited to arugula, beet greens, bok choy, chicory, Chinese cabbage, collard greens, dandelion greens, endive, kale, mustard greens, romaine lettuce, spinach, Swiss chard, turnip greens, and watercress.

Each of these greens has its own history, and space does not permit us to explore them. As an example, however, we know that the ancient Greeks grew kale and collards, and that spinach originated in the Middle East and was brought to Spain between 800 and 1200 A.D. Greens have a history of medicinal use as well: dandelion greens, for example, have been highly regarded for their ability to reduce water retention and aid in digestive disorders, while beet greens were used by the ancient Romans to treat wounds.

NUTRITIONAL VALUE—BEET GREENS
1 cup cooked
Calories: 39
Fiber: 4.2 g, 13%

Iron: 2.7 mg, 33% DRI
Magnesium: 98 mg, 23% DRI
Potassium: 1309 mg, 28% DRI
Riboflavin: 0.4 mg, 31% DRI
Vitamin A: 11,022 IU, 367% DRI
Vitamin C: 36 mg, 40% DRI

NUTRITIONAL VALUE—KALE
1 cup chopped, cooked
Calories: 36
Fiber: 2.6 g, 8%
Calcium: 94 mg
Iron: 1.17 mg, 14% DRI
Potassium: 296 mg, 6% DRI
Vitamin A: 17,707 IU, 590% DRI
Vitamin C: 53 mg, 59% DRI

NUTRITIONAL VALUE—SPINACH
1 cup chopped, cooked
Calories: 44
Fiber: 4.3 g, 13%
Calcium: 245 mg
Folic acid: 263 mcg, 66% DRI
Iron: 6.4 mg, 79% DRI
Magnesium: 157 mg, 37% DRI
Potassium: 839 mg, 18% DRI
Vitamin A: 18,866 IU, 628% DRI
Vitamin C: 17.6 mg, 20% DRI

NUTRITIONAL VALUE—SWISS CHARD
1 cup chopped, cooked
Calories: 35
Calcium: 102 mg

Fiber: 3.7 g, 12%
Iron: 3.95 mg, 49% DRI
Magnesium: 150 mg, 36% DRI

Why Greens Are Heart-Healthy

Overall, leafy green vegetables are a powerhouse of nutrients that are good for the heart. Vying for the top of the list are carotenes, including beta-carotene, lutein, and zeaxanthin. Then there are minerals such as potassium, magnesium, and calcium. And we must not forget vitamin C and its antioxidant properties. Here are some findings by the experts.

- The results of a meta-analysis published in 2008 reported that an increase in dietary intake of the antioxidants beta-carotene and vitamins C and E offer protection against coronary heart disease.

- Numerous studies have shown that carotenoids such as lutein, zeaxanthin, and beta-carotene, all found in leafy green vegetables, provide protection against cardiovascular disease.

- A study in which rats were fed a 20 percent lettuce diet for three weeks resulted in a decrease in cholesterol levels and in the LDL/HDL ratio. The lettuce diet also improved the levels of antioxidants (vitamins C and E, carotenoids). Therefore regular consumption of lettuce appears to help protect against cardiovascular diseases.

RECIPE

This recipe is for all you pasta lovers who may have been disappointed that pasta isn't among the heart-healthy foods. But when we combine pasta with greens, the result is a delicious and nutritious entrée that everyone can enjoy. Just don't tell your kids that it's good for them!

Greens and Pasta
Serves 4–6
3 lbs dandelion, mustard, or turnip greens
1 lb pasta of your choice (whole grain preferred)
1 tsp salt
4 cloves garlic, minced
1/8 cup virgin olive oil
Black pepper and salt, to taste
Pinch dried red pepper flakes

In a large pot, bring 2 to 3 quarts of water and the salt to a boil. In the meantime, trim and wash the greens and cut them into 1-inch pieces. When the water comes to a boil, add the greens and cook until they are nearly tender but still bright green, 8 to 10 minutes. Remove the greens with a slotted spoon and place them in a large bowl of cold water. Add the pasta to the pot of water and cook until done. While the pasta is cooking, squeeze the greens to remove as much water as possible. In a large skillet, heat the olive oil over medium-high heat. Add the garlic and stir until it begins to brown. Add the pepper flakes and drained greens and stir together for about 2 minutes. Drain the pasta and add to the cooked greens. Toss well and season with pepper and salt. Serve immediately.

GREEN TEA

Although we may think of green tea as a novelty or as just an alternative to black tea, originally all the tea that people consumed was green. Tea has been used in China as a beverage—often for medicinal purposes—for about 5,000 years. The earliest known reference to the use of tea for health purposes is 2737 B.C.

Originally tea was reserved for the wealthy and elite. It wasn't until the fall of the Mongolian empire in 1368 A.D. that the general population was able to enjoy the beverage as well. When China was a sea power from 1405 until 1433, green tea was credited with warding off scurvy for seamen. If the European sailors about 100 years later had known this, they might have been able to prevent many deaths from the disease.

Black and oolong teas came into popularity and significant production around 1650 A.D. in China. Because these teas are processed, they have a much longer shelf life than green tea and thus they were suitable for export to Europe and other markets.

Tea drinking didn't become popular in the United States until about 1945, when it was introduced from Europe as part of the worldwide tea trade and through Chinese restaurants that opened in the States. It was black tea, however, that made its debut. Today, green tea is still an acquired taste for many Americans.

NUTRITIONAL VALUE—GREEN TEA

If you look at a nutritional label on a green tea product, you won't see any of the traditional information. But green tea does contain more than 450 organic compounds that are important for health, including minimal amounts of some minerals, protein, amino acids, vitamins, and of course, significant levels of polyphenols, including epigallocatechin gallate (EGCG) and epigallocatechin (EGC).

Why Green Tea Is Heart-Healthy

The main health benefits from green tea are due to its high content of flavonoids, especially a group called catechins. These powerful antioxidants have been shown to be more potent than vitamins C and E in the fight against free-radical damage to cells. Is green tea better than black? When it comes to polyphenols, it is: Green tea contains 30 to 40 percent polyphenols, while black tea contains 3 to 10 percent. Oolong tea falls somewhere in between green and black tea. The four main polyphenols found in fresh tea leaves are epigallocatechin gallate (EGCG), epigallocatechin (EGC), epicatechin gallate (ECG), and epicatechin (EC).

Here's why green tea is good for the heart:

- The antioxidants in green tea help block the oxidation of low-density lipoprotein (LDL, "bad") cholesterol, raise levels of high-density lipoprotein (HDL, "good") cholesterol, and improve functioning of the arteries.

- A recent study from Greece shows that regular consumption of green tea may improve the function of the cells that line the walls of blood vessels (endothelial cells), which in turn boosts heart health.

- Green tea extract can reduce blood pressure and cholesterol, according to a recent multi-center study published in *Nutrition*. A randomized, double-blind, placebo-controlled study found that green extract reduced oxidative stress, systolic and diastolic blood pressures by 5 and 4 mmHg, respectively, and total cholesterol levels by 10 mg/dL. It also decreased a marker of chronic inflammation. All of these are risk factors for cardiovascular disease.

• Both animal studies and human studies show that green tea can help reduce weight, and obesity is a risk factor for heart disease. Generally, the studies show that the catechin antioxidants help reduce body fat and promote fat burning.

RECIPE

When making green tea, use 1 teaspoon of loose tea leaves or a standard tea bag and steep it in hot, but not boiling, water for 2 minutes. Use of boiling water and longer steeping times cause the tea to become bitter and also reduce the nutritional value. With that in mind, here's a green tea smoothie recipe. It makes about 2½ cups.

Green Tea Smoothie
Serves one
1½ cups frozen berries—your choice
¾ cup fat-free soy milk or plain yogurt
½ cup brewed green tea
1 peeled banana, frozen
¼ cup pomegranate juice

Place all the ingredients into a blender and blend until smooth. Serve immediately.

KIWI

The kiwi is a native of China, where it was known as Yang Tao. This fuzzy fruit was carried to New Zealand by missionaries in the early twentieth century, where it was eventually renamed Chinese gooseberries. Kiwi didn't reach the United States until 1961, when a produce distributor thought the strange fruit would be a welcome addition to the fruit scene in the States. When she finally arranged to import Chinese gooseberries into the United States, she changed the name to kiwifruit, named in honor of the kiwi, the native bird of New Zealand. Today, the leading commercial producers of kiwifruit are Italy, New Zealand, Chile, France, Japan, and the United States.

NUTRITIONAL VALUE—KIWI, RAW
1 cup
Calories: 108
Fiber: 5.3 mg, 17%
Calcium: 60 mg
Folic acid: 44 mcg, 11% DRI
Potassium: 552 mg, 12% DRI
Vitamin C: 164 mg, 182% DRI

Why Kiwi Is Heart-Healthy
Along with its excellent levels of vitamin C, kiwi contains a variety of phytonutrients, including lutein and zeaxanthin, which promote heart and overall health. Here are some reasons why.

- In a 2004 study, researchers evaluated the impact of kiwi on lipids and platelets in healthy volunteers. They found that participants who ate

2 to 3 kiwi daily for 28 days reduced their platelet aggregation response (which is an indication of blood clot formation) by 18 percent and their triglyceride levels by 15 percent compared to volunteers who did not eat kiwi. These benefits are credited to the vitamin C, polyphenols, vitamin E, magnesium, potassium, and copper found in kiwi.

- Kiwi is a very good source of fiber. Research shows that diets that contain lots of fiber can lower cholesterol levels, which in turn may reduce the risk of heart disease, heart attack, and stroke. Fiber also helps keep blood sugar levels low, an important benefit for people who have diabetes, who are at high risk of heart disease.

RECIPE

Kiwi is a real treat just on its own—just slice, peel, and eat. For a refreshing kiwi beverage, try the following.

Kiwi Blend
Serves 2
2 kiwifruit
1 ripe banana
1 tsp lime juice
1/2 tsp grated lime zest
1 cup fat-free milk
1/4 cup fat-free plain yogurt

Peel the kiwi and banana and cut into chunks. Place the fruit, lime juice, and zest in a blender or food processor and process until blended. Add the milk and yogurt and process for 5 to 10 seconds. Pour into glasses and serve.

LENTILS

Lentils are legumes that have been on the human menu since prehistoric times. Archaeologists have found evidence of lentil seeds in the Middle East dating back 8,000 years. Traditionally lentils have been eaten with wheat and barley. Hippocrates prescribed lentils for his patients who had liver disorders.

Lentils were introduced into India before the first century A.D., and they are still highly regarded in that country as a staple in the diet. In Catholic countries, lentils have been used during Lent as a protein source instead of meat. The main commercial producers of lentils today include India, Canada, Turkey, China, and Syria.

NUTRITIONAL VALUE—LENTILS, COOKED

$^1/_2$ cup
Calories: 115
Fiber: 7.8 g, 24%
Calcium: 19 mg
Folic acid: 179 mcg, 45% DRI
Iron: 3.3 mg, 41% DRI
Potassium: 365 mg, 8% DRI
Thiamin: 0.17 mg, 14% DRI
Vitamin B_6: 0.17 mg, 10% DRI
Zinc: 1.2 mg, 11% DRI

Why Lentils Are Heart-Healthy

The often-neglected lentil is a very nutritious food, providing high levels of protein, fiber, B vitamins, and minerals with nearly no fat. Specifically, it offers several advantages when it comes to heart health.

- Lentils are an especially good source of fiber, which captures cholesterol and transports it out of the body. In a study published in the *Archives of Internal Medicine,* researchers verified that eating foods high in fiber, such as lentils, helps prevent heart disease. Participants who ate the most fiber (21 grams daily) had 12 percent less coronary heart disease and 11 percent less cardiovascular disease, compared to those who ate the least (5 grams daily).

- In the Seven Countries Study, investigators evaluated the food patterns and risk of death from coronary heart disease in more than 16,000 middle-aged men for 25 years. The food patterns included higher consumption of vegetables, legumes, fish, and wine in Southern Europe; higher consumption of cereals, soy, and fish in Japan; higher consumption of dairy foods in Northern Europe; and higher consumption of meat in the United States. When the researchers analyzed all the data, they noted that legumes were associated with a 82 percent reduced risk in coronary heart disease.

- The magnesium in lentils helps relax blood vessels, which improves the flow of oxygen, blood, and nutrients. A magnesium deficiency is associated with injury to the heart muscle and heart attack.

• Lentils contain a good amount of folic acid. This B vitamin, along with vitamins B_6 and B_{12}, help reduce levels of homocysteine, an amino acid that can damage artery walls and increase the risk for heart disease.

RECIPE

There's nothing like a bowl of hearty soup on a cold day, and lentil soup certainly fits the bill. Here's a recipe that is easy to prepare and tastes even better left over. So make a big pot!

Lentil Soup
Serves 6 to 8
2 cups lentils, rinsed
1 Tbs olive oil
1 large onion, chopped
1 bell pepper, chopped
1 28-oz can crushed tomatoes, no salt
8 cups water
3 cups greens, finely chopped
1 tsp salt

Bring 6 cups of water to a boil, add the lentils, and cook for about 20 minutes or until tender. Drain and set aside. Heat the oil in a heavy soup pot and add the onion, pepper, and salt and sauté until tender. Stir in the tomatoes, lentils, and 2 cups of water and bring the soup to a simmer. Stir in the greens and stir for 1 to 2 minutes. Season as desired, and serve.

MANGO

The mango we know and love today is a sweeter, much better-tasting version of the wild mango that originated in the Himalayas of Burma and India before 4000 B.C. Fortunately, the Indians began cultivating the fruit around 2000 B.C. or earlier, which resulted in the superior tropical fruit of today. The mango made its journey from southern India to Africa in the sixteenth century with Portuguese explorers. It was introduced to Brazil and the West Indies in the eighteenth century and to Florida in the nineteenth century.

Mangoes are members of the cashew family and can range in size from two to 10 inches. Although there are more than 400 varieties of mango around the world, the two most widely available ones are the Kent (green with a red blush and a very sweet flavor) and Keitt (green with a mild sweet flavor). Others include the Tommy Atkins and the Haden. The top producers of mango are India, Pakistan, Puerto Rico, Mexico, Brazil, Israel, South Africa, and Peru.

NUTRITIONAL VALUE—MANGO

1 cup slices
Calories: 107
Fiber: 3 g, 9%
Potassium: 257 mg, 5% DRI
Vitamin A: 1,262 IU, 42% DRI
Vitamin C: 46 mg, 51% DRI

Why Mango Is Heart-Healthy

Like many tropical fruits, mangoes are rich sources of antioxidants. Mangoes also harbor heart-healthy phenolic compounds, including quercetin, isoquercitfin, astragalin, fisetin, gallic acid, and methylgallat. Here's what the experts say.

- Many studies show that the antioxidants vitamins A and C, which are found in mangoes, play an important role in helping prevent heart disease. These nutrients help stop free radical damage to the heart, and prevent the accumulation of plaque on the walls of the arteries, which can hinder blood flow and cause stroke and heart attack.

- A study from the Boston University School of Medicine found that the cardiovascular benefits associated with polyphenol flavonoids seems to be related to their ability to improve endothelial function, which is critical for heart health, and to inhibit the accumulation of platelets, which plays a central role in coronary conditions such as myocardial infarction and unstable angina.

- Mango is a good source of potassium, a mineral that is crucial for cardiovascular health, as it is necessary to transmit electrical signals in the heart. If you take diuretics, you may have low potassium levels, which can cause a disruption in the electrical impulses and cause irregular heartbeat.

- A recent study published in the *British Journal of Nutrition* reported that quercetin, which is found in mangoes, reduces systolic blood pressure and low-density lipoprotein cholesterol and that the phytonutrient may provide protection against cardiovascular disease.

RECIPE

Mangoes are delicious just as they are: just peel, slice, and eat. But if you want a different treat, try the Frozen Mango Magic. Double up on the recipe and keep extra in your freezer!

Frozen Mango Magic
2 Tbs honey
2 tsp chopped fresh ginger
1 egg, separated
Pinch of salt
Pinch of cream of tartar
2 Tbs sugar
2 cups nonfat plain yogurt
2 medium mangoes

Peel, pit, and chop the mangoes. Puree with the honey and ginger in a food processor or blender. Bring the puree to a boil in a saucepan. Gradually whisk in a beaten egg yolk, then set it aside to cool. Beat the egg white with salt and cream of tartar until peaks form. Gradually beat in the sugar until stiff peaks form. Stir the yogurt into the mango mixture and then fold in the egg white. Spread the mixture into a shallow metal pan and freeze until firm.

OATMEAL

The oats that find their way into your breakfast cereal or cookies can trace their roots from a wild red oat that originated in Asia. Even before people used oats for food, they recognized the medicinal value of this widely grown crop. Oats *(Avena sativa)* were a dietary staple for people in Scotland, Great Britain, Germany, and the Scandinavian countries. Scottish settlers brought oats to North America in the early seventeenth century. Today, the United States, Russia, Poland, and Finland are major producers of oats.

Oats undergo various processing methods to produce the different types available on the market. Although oats are hulled, this does not eliminate the nutritious bran and germ that help make oats so good for you. The main types of oats you can find in supermarkets include:

- **Oat bran.** The outer layer of the grain that is found under the hull. It is sold as a separate product that can be cooked as a hot cereal or added to recipes.

- **Oat groats.** The unflattened kernels that are used for cereal or stuffing.

- **Steel-cut.** This process gives the oats a dense and chewy texture.

- **Old-fashioned oats.** These oats are steamed and rolled to give them a flat shape.

- **Quick-cooking oats.** These are processed like the old-fashioned variety except they are finely cut before they are rolled.

- **Instant oatmeal.** The oats are partially cooked and then rolled very thin.

NUTRITIONAL VALUE—OATMEAL

1 cup cooked, instant, plain

Calories: 159

Fiber: 4 g, 13%

Calcium: 187 mg

Iron: 14 mg, 172% DRI

Thiamin: 0.6 mg, 50% DRI

Riboflavin: 0.5 mg, 38% DRI

Niacin: 7.0 mg, 44% DRI

Vitamin B_6: 0.7, 41% DRI

Folic acid: 103 mcg, 26% DRI

Why Oats Are Heart-Healthy

Fiber is usually the first thing that comes to mind whenever people talk about the heart-healthy attributes of oats and oatmeal, and they are right. But oats also bring a few other benefits to the table.

• When it comes to fiber, let's do the math. Studies show that just 3 grams of soluble oat fiber consumed daily (the amount found in an 8-ounce serving of oatmeal) can reduce total cholesterol by 8 to 23 percent. Because each 1 percent drop in serum cholesterol translates to a 2 percent decrease in the risk of developing heart disease, eating oatmeal is definitely a good decision. One study that defined just how good oats are for the heart was published in the *Archives of Internal Medicine*. The nineteen-year study involved nearly 10,000 adults. Those who ate 21 grams of fiber daily had 12 percent less coronary heart disease and 11 percent less cardiovascular disease compared with adults who ate 5 grams daily.

- Oats contain antioxidants called avenanthramides, which are unique to this grain. A study in lab animals found that avenanthramides help prevent damage from free radicals (oxidation), which in turn reduces the risk of cardiovascular disease. A study of avenanthramides in human arterial cells found that the antioxidants suppressed the production of several types of molecules involved in the development of atherosclerosis, as well as the secretion of pro-inflammatory cytokines, which are also involved in heart disease. In both studies, the researchers found that the addition of vitamin C enhances the benefits of avenanthramides.

- The Physicians Health Study, which followed 21,376 participants over nearly 20 years, found that men who consumed a bowl of whole grain cereal daily, like oats, had a 29 percent lower risk of heart failure than those who did not.

- Postmenopausal women with cardiovascular disease who consumed whole grains such as oats at least six times per week experienced slowed progression of atherosclerosis (the accumulation of plaque in the blood vessels) and less progression in stenosis (narrowing of the diameter of the arteries).

- Oats contain a phytochemical called lignans, which are converted by bacteria in the intestinal tract into enterolactone, which is believed to protect against heart disease.

RECIPE

What better way to begin your day than with a bowl of oatmeal? And not just any oatmeal, but a cereal that is colorful, nutritious, and tastes great. Here's just one of many ways to enjoy oats.

Almond Blueberry Oatmeal
Serves 1
1 cup water
¼ cup steel cut oats (you can use any kind you like)
⅓ cup fresh blueberries (or berry of your choice)
¼ cup non-fat milk
1 Tbs chopped almonds
1 tsp ground flaxseed

Bring 1 cup of water to a boil and add the oats. Allow the oats to boil for about 5 minutes. Reduce heat to a simmer and cook for 20–25 minutes, stirring occasionally. Turn off the heat and add the remaining ingredients. You can garnish with additional berries.

OLIVE OIL

Olive trees *(Olea europaea)* have been around since ancient times, and olives are among the oldest foods known to man. Experts believe olive oil was first made around 3000 B.C. and probably originated in the Mediterranean region. Olives were transported to America by Portuguese and Spanish explorers during the fifteenth and sixteenth centuries and were embraced by the Franciscan missionaries in California in the late eighteenth century. Olive oil did not gain great popularity in the United States until the past few decades when it was discovered that the oil is high in monounsaturated fat, which helps reduce the risk of heart disease and other serious conditions.

Most commercial production of olive oil is done in the Mediterranean in countries such as Spain, Italy, Portugal, Turkey, and Greece. The olive oil that they produce is available in a range of grades, which reflect how much the oil has been processed. Here are what some of the terms mean.

- Extra-virgin means the oil is unrefined and is derived from the first pressing of the olives. It is the highest grade and has the most delicate taste of all grades of olive oil. It is recommended for salad dressings and dipping.

- Virgin olive oil is also the product of the first pressing, but it has a higher acidity level than extra virgin oil. The deciding factor is the amount of olelic acid, which indicates overall acidity: Virgin oil can contain up to 2% oleic acid, while extra virgin contains only up to 0.8% oleic acid.

- Ordinary olive oil can contain up to 3.3% olelic acid. This is the grade of olive oil that some use for cooking because it has a higher smoke temperature than virgin and extra-virgin olive oils.

- Cold-pressed means that minimal heat was used when the olives were mechanically pressed to make oil.

NUTRITIONAL VALUE—OLIVE OIL
1 tablespoon
Calories: 119

Total fat: 13.5 mg
Monounsaturated fat: 9.9 mg

Why Olive Oil Is Heart-Healthy

Olive oil is a staple in the Mediterranean diet, and experts believe it is one of the main reasons why this diet approach is so heart-healthy. Scores of studies have been done on the merits of olive oil for heart-related conditions, and just a few of them are noted here.

- The CARDIO2000 study, which involved 700 men and 148 women who had coronary heart disease and 1,078 healthy controls, found that exclusive use of olive oil (i.e., participants did not use soy, corn, sunflower, or any other kind of oil) was associated with a 47 percent lower risk of having coronary heart disease.

- A recent study found that the polyphenolic compounds present in olive oil, including oleuropein, prevent monocyte cells from sticking to the blood vessel lining, a process that leads to atherosclerosis.

- Research results published in the *Journal of Agriculture and Food Chemistry* show that the phenols in olive oil, such as protocatechuic acid and oleuropein, help prevent the oxidation of LDL, a process that leads to atherosclerosis. The phenols also inhibit the production of damaging free radicals and restore to normal levels two critical enzymes—glutathione reductase and glutathione peroxidase—which disarm free radicals. All of these activities protect the heart.

- In November 2004, the Food and Drug Administration (FDA) allowed olive oil producers to place a claim on their products concerning "the benefits on the risk of coronary heart disease of eating about two tablespoons (23 g) of olive oil daily, due to the monounsaturated fat (MUFA) in olive oil."

- A Spanish study found that the oleic acid found in olive oil is responsible for the oil's ability to lower high blood pressure. Oleic acid is more resistant to free radical or oxidative damage.

- Olive oil reduces inflammation, which protects the lining of the blood vessels (endothelium), which in turn allows them to relax and dilate without raising blood pressure. The anti-inflammatory benefits of olive oil also help prevent platelets from clumping together and forming blood clots, which can result in heart attack or stroke.

RECIPE

Olive oil is the perfect base for a good salad dressing, so we offer a suggestion here that can be used not only on salads but on just any of your favorite vegetables.

Olive Oil and Lemon Dressing
Makes about 1½ cups
1 cup fresh lemon juice

$1/2$ cup extra virgin olive oil
8 cloves garlic, minced
$1/2$ tsp black pepper
2 tsp salt
1 tsp dried dill

Combine all ingredients in a shaker bottle and shake vigorously.

ONIONS

Onions *(Allium cepa)* have been an important part of the diet for more than five thousand years. This member of the lily family is a native to the Middle East and Asia. In ancient times onions were especially valued by the Egyptians, who placed them in the tombs of their kings and used them to pay the builders of the Pyramids. The medicinal value of onions was recognized as early as the sixth century, when people in India used them for coughs and breathing problems.

There are more than 600 species of *Allium*, and they can be found throughout Europe, North America, Northern Africa, and Asia. Onions and other *Allium* vegetables (e.g., scallions, leeks, garlic) are characterized by various sulfur compounds, which give them their odor and their ability to make your eyes water.

Although you may not think of onions as a breakfast food, this vegetable was a common menu item for the first meal of the day in some European countries centuries ago. Columbus brought onions to the West Indies, and eventually they were cultivated throughout the Western Hemisphere. The leading producers of onions today include China, India, the United States, Russia, and Spain.

NUTRITIONAL VALUE—ONIONS, SWEET, RAW
One medium
Calories: 106
Fiber: 3 g, 9%
Calcium: 66 mg
Folic acid: 76 mcg, 19% DRI
Potassium: 394 mg, 8% DRI
Vitamin B$_6$: 0.43 mg, 25% DRI

NUTRITIONAL VALUE—SCALLIONS, RAW
1 cup chopped (includes bulbs)
Calories: 32
Fiber: 2.6 g, 8%
Calcium: 72 mg
Folic acid: 64 mcg, 16% DRI
Iron: 1.48 mg, 18% DRI
Potassium: 276 mg, 6% DRI
Vitamin A: 997 IU, 33% DRI

Why Onions Are Heart-Healthy

Onions are a major source of the phytonutrients called phenols and flavonoids, which have been shown to protect against cardiovascular disease and cancer. When it comes to these nutrients, not all onions are created equal. Here is what the research says.

- According to research published in the *Journal of Agricultural and Food Chemistry* (November 2004), certain onions provide more heart-healthy compounds than others. The investigators evaluated shallots and 10 other types of onions (e.g., Western Yellow, Western White, Vidalia, and more). For maximum antioxidant power, shallots topped the list while Vidalia was at the bottom. Shallots also had the most phenols, again leaving Vidalia at the end of the list. For the most flavonoids, Western Yellow topped the list, with 11 times the amount found in the onion with the lowest content, Western White.

• Regular consumption of onions can reduce cholesterol and blood pressure levels, both of which help prevent diabetic heart disease and atherosclerosis and reduce the risk of stroke and heart attack. Experts believe these benefits can be credited to the sulfur compounds in onions, as well as their good levels of vitamin B_6 and chromium.

• Onions are an especially rich source of flavonoids, which, in a meta-analysis of seven prospective studies, were found to significantly reduce the risk of heart disease. More than 100,000 people participated in these studies, which noted that individuals whose diets frequently included onions, tea, apples, and broccoli (all rich sources of flavonoids) enjoyed this lower risk of heart disease.

• Onions contain natural anti-clotting substances, which help reduce the risk of stroke and heart attack.

RECIPE

Onions come in a range of colors and degrees of pungency, as well as nutritional value. This recipe calls for sweet onions and scallions, although you could use more than one type to fulfill the "4 large sweet onion" portion.

Baked Onions and Potatoes
Serves 4–6
4 potatoes (about 1¹/₂ lbs)
4 large sweet onions
¹/₂ cup finely chopped scallions
³/₄ cup vegetable broth, salt-free
2 tsp dried tarragon
Salt and pepper to taste

Cut the potatoes and onions into 8 wedges each. Place the wedges in a ¹/₂-inch deep baking pan. Combine the broth and tarragon and pour over the vegetables. Season with salt and pepper to taste. Roast in a 450°F oven for 20 minutes.

ORANGES

Thousands of years ago, the predecessor of today's sweet oranges grew wild in China and possibly also in India and Myanmar. The wild orange was sour, although somewhere along the line sweeter varieties were cultivated. The Chinese were likely the first to cultivate oranges beginning around 2500 B.C. Oranges didn't make their way to the Romans and to North Africa until about the first century A.D. The Moors brought oranges to southern Spain in the eighth or ninth century, after which they spread to Italy.

Christopher Columbus brought orange seeds or trees with him when he traveled to the island of Hispaniola in the Caribbean. The Spanish brought oranges to St.

Augustine, Florida, in 1565, where they quickly became popular. Oranges remain a major crop in Florida today, although the world's leading producer of oranges is Brazil, which provides 50 percent of the world's orange juice and 80 percent of the world's trade in concentrated orange juice.

NUTRITIONAL VALUE—ORANGES
One large (3" diameter), raw without peel
Calories: 86
Fiber: 4.4 g, 14%
Calcium: 74 mg, 82% DRI
Potassium: 333 mg, 7% DRI
Vitamin C: 98 mg, 108% DRI

Why Oranges Are Heart-Healthy
Most people think of vitamin C whenever oranges are mentioned, and it's true that these citrus wonders are an excellent source of this potent antioxidant. Vitamin C is not the only reason oranges are good for the cardiovascular system; they also contain more than 170 different phytonutrients and more than 60 flavonoids. However, we will begin our explanation of the heart-healthy virtues of oranges with vitamin C.

- Because vitamin C can neutralize free radicals, it helps prevent the oxidation of cholesterol, which in turn prevents plaque from accumulating on the walls of your arteries.

- Oranges contain various phytonutrients, including the flavonoids hesperetin and naringenin; anthocyanins; hydroxycinnamic acids; and many polyphenols. While all of these phytonutrients work in synergy with vitamin C, research has shown that one in particular, herperidin, reduces both cholesterol and high blood pressure, and also is an anti-inflammatory. Since herperidin is found only in the inner white pulp and peel of oranges, it is recommended that you eat at least some of the white pulp when enjoying an orange.

• A large U.S. study found that one extra serving of citrus fruit daily can reduce the risk of stroke by up to 19 percent. The study was part of a larger research effort called Commonwealth Scientific and Industrial Research (CSIRO), which reviewed 48 studies that show a diet rich in citrus provides significant protection against some cancers and other medical conditions.

• The CSIRO also reported that consuming citrus also protects against overweight and obesity, which increase the risk of heart disease, high blood pressure, and stroke.

• The World Health Organization, in its report "Diet Nutrition and the Prevention of Chronic Disease," found that a diet that features citrus protects against cardiovascular disease because the fruit contains folic acid, potassium, vitamin C, carotenoids, and flavonoids.

• A substance in oranges called limonin appears to reduce cholesterol levels in laboratory studies.

• Compounds called polymethoxylated flavones
  (PMFs), which are found in orange peels and in
  small amounts in the fruit itself, seem to reduce
  cholesterol in lab animals. Rats with high cholesterol who were given PMFs had a 19 to 27 percent decrease in total cholesterol. The most
  common PMFs are tangeretin and nobiletin. Researchers believe PMFs work like statins, which
  inhibit the synthesis of cholesterol inside the
  liver.

• Oranges are also a good source of fiber, which
  reduces high cholesterol levels and helps keep
  blood sugar levels under control.

RECIPE
The best way to reap the benefits of oranges is to eat them
raw. Here's a delicious, if slightly unusual, way to enjoy
them.

Orange and Red Salad
Serves 2
2 large oranges, peeled, seeded, and sectioned
1/4 cup chopped red onion
1/4 cup chopped red bell pepper
6 medium black olives, chopped
1 tsp olive oil

*Combine all ingredients in a bowl and mix well. Chill
until ready to serve.*

PAPAYA

They are sweet and have a buttery consistency and a musky taste. They are papaya, a tropical fruit with orange flesh that has been called "the fruit of the angels." Papayas are indigenous to Central America, where the natives have long honored them. The fruit is perhaps best known for the enzyme that it contains called papain, which helps digest proteins. This substance makes it valued as a digestive aid.

Papayas were brought to India, Africa, and the Philippines by Portuguese and Spanish explorers during the 1500s. They didn't make their way to the United States until the 1900s, when they were introduced to Florida, probably from the Bahamas. Today the largest U.S. producer of papaya is Hawaii. The fruit is also grown in Mexico, Puerto Rico, and other tropical regions.

Papayas (also called paw-paws) come in two varieties: solo and Mexican. Solo papaya weigh about 1 pound and are green-yellow on the outside. Mexican papayas are larger; they can weigh up to 10 pounds. Less sweet than the solo variety, they tend to be greener on the outside.

NUTRITIONAL VALUE—PAPAYA

1 cup cubes
Calories: 55
Fiber: 2.5 g, 8%
Calcium: 34 mg
Folic acid: 53 mcg, 13% DRI
Potassium: 360 mg, 8% DRI
Vitamin A: 1,532 IU, 51% DRI
Vitamin C: 87 mg, 97% DRI

Why Papaya Is Heart-Healthy

As a tropical fruit, papayas are a rich source of antioxidants and phytonutrients, which can have beneficial effects on the heart. Here are a few reasons why papayas are a good choice to include in your diet.

• Papayas are an excellent source of vitamin C and a good source of vitamins E and A, all potent antioxidants. Antioxidants help prevent the oxidation of cholesterol, and thus this sticky substance cannot accumulate on the inside walls of blood vessels and impede blood flow and result in stroke or heart attack.

• Papayas contain a compound called paraoxonase, an enzyme that works with vitamins C and E to inhibit the oxidation of LDL cholesterol and HDL cholesterol.

• The fiber content of papayas is helpful in lowering cholesterol levels.

• As a source of folic acid, papayas help convert the heart-damaging amino acid called homocysteine into a benign amino acid such as methionine or cysteine.

• Papaya contains enzymes called papain and chymopapain, which can reduce inflammation. Since heart disease involves inflammation, papaya may provide some benefit in this regard as well.

RECIPE

This easy recipe combines papaya and another delicious fruit, pears.

Poached Papaya
Serves 4
1 large ripe papaya
1 large pear
1/2 cup unsweetened orange juice
1 tsp shredded lemon or lime peel
1/4 tsp ground nutmeg
1 tsp cornstarch
1 tsp lemon or lime juice

Cut the papaya in half lengthwise, remove the peel and seeds, and cut the pulp into cubes. Halve and core the pear and cut into thin slices.

In a medium skillet, combine the orange juice, peel, and nutmeg. Add the cut-up fruit and bring the mixture to a boil. Reduce heat, cover and simmer for 3 to 5 minutes or until the pear is tender. Remove the fruit from the skillet with a slotted spoon and place in a bowl. Put the lime or lemon juice and cornstarch into a small cup, stir well, and add it to the orange juice mixture, stirring continuously until the mixture thickens. Cook the mixture for about 2 additional minutes and pour it over the fruit. Serve warm or cool.

PLUMS

Few people realize the vast array of plums (*Prunus domestica*) that is available. The six main categories of plums—Japanese, American, Damson, Ornamental, Wild, and European—encompass more than 2,000 varieties. Although many plums are round, they can also be heart-shaped or oval. Colors range from red to purple, blue-black, green, amber, or yellow, and their flesh can be yellow, green, pink, or orange.

European plums may have been discovered near the Caspian Sea about two thousand years ago. They were introduced to the United States by the Pilgrims in the seventeenth century. Japanese plums were first found in China, but they were mostly cultivated and developed in Japan. The Japanese varieties did not make their way into the United States until the late nineteenth century. Today they are the most commonly eaten fresh plum.

The main producers of plums today are the United States, Russia, China, and Romania. Plums are enjoyed both fresh and dried, as prunes. We discuss both fresh and dried plums in this entry.

NUTRITIONAL VALUE—PLUMS, FRESH
Two 2⅛" fruits
Calories: 61
Fiber: 1.8 g, 6%
Potassium: 207 mg, 4% DRI
Vitamin A: 455 IU, 15% DRI
Vitamin C: 12.5 mg, 14% DRI

NUTRITIONAL VALUE—PLUMS, DRIED (PRUNES)
½ cup
Calories: 209
Fiber: 6.2 g, 19%
Calcium: 37 mg
Iron: 0.81 mg, 10% DRI
Niacin: 1.6 mg, 10% DRI

Potassium: 637 mg, 14% DRI
Vitamin A: 679 IU, 23% DRI

Why Plums Are Heart-Healthy

Plums and prunes contain some potent phytonutrients, including the phenols neochlorogenic and chlorogenic acid. These phenols act as antioxidants and are helpful in heart health. Along with phenols, plums offer some other advantages for the heart.

- The phenols in plums are effective in neutralizing a potent radical called superoxide anion radical, as well as preventing the oxidation of cholesterol and triglycerides, which contribute to the development of heart disease.

- A January 2009 study published in the *British Journal of Nutrition* suggests that eating prunes can slow down the development of atherosclerosis. One of the study's authors noted that the findings reinforced the idea that eating fruit, and especially dried plums, can help prevent heart disease.

- Plums are a good source of vitamin C, which helps to protect against the oxidation of cholesterol by free radicals. Because oxidized cholesterol is the type that accumulates in the arteries and damages the blood vessels, vitamin C is essential for people who have diabetic heart disease or atherosclerosis.

- Dried plums provide a very good source of fiber, which helps in the control of high cholesterol.

RECIPE

Fresh plums are always a convenient and sweet treat, as are dried plums, yet dried plums (which used to be called prunes; the name was changed for marketing purposes) still have an image problem. This recipe may change that.

Dried Plum Compote
Serves 6
6 oranges
1/2 cup dried plums, quartered
1/2 cup water
2 Tbs sugar
1/4 cup dried cranberries
1/4 cup crushed walnuts
1/4 tsp ground cinnamon

Peel and deseed the oranges and cut the oranges cross-wise into 1/2-inch slices. Arrange the orange slices and dried plums in a bowl. In a saucepan, simmer the water and sugar until the sugar dissolves. Remove from the heat and cool. Pour it over the oranges and dried plums. Cover and refrigerate for 30 minutes or longer. Before serving, garnish with cranberries, walnuts, and cinnamon.

POMEGRANATE

Also known as the "apple of many seeds," pomegranates have been around since ancient times. The first cultivated pomegranates appeared more than four thousand years ago near the Tigris and Euphrates in what is modern day Iraq. Pomegranates were introduced to the Chinese in the second century B.C., and the fruit is mentioned in the Old Testament in several places. Some people even believe that the "apple of many seeds" was the apple in the Garden of Eden.

Because the pomegranate has a hard shell, it travels well and protects the water (it consists of about 80 percent water) and seeds inside. The Spanish transported it to Mexico in the 1500s and to California about a century later. Yet for all its hardiness, the pomegranate did not become popular in the United States mostly because it is not an easy fruit to eat. In recent years, however, research has uncovered many health advantages of pomegranates, and more people are taking a second look at the fruit and its juice.

NUTRITIONAL VALUE—POMEGRANATE, RAW
One 4" fruit
Calories: 234
Fiber: 11.3 g, 35%
Calcium: 28 mg
Folic acid: 107 mcg, 27% DRI
Potassium: 666 mg, 14% DRI
Vitamin C: 29 mg, 32% DRI

NUTRITIONAL VALUE—POMEGRANATE JUICE
4 ounces
Calories: 67
Folic acid: 30 mcg, 8% DRI
Potassium: 266 mg, 6% DRI

Why Pomegranates Are Heart-Healthy

Pomegranates are rich in antioxidants, including polyphenols such as tannins and anthyocyanins. In fact, ounce for ounce, they have about three times more free-radical fighting power than green tea or red wine. The antioxidants in pomegranates have been shown to benefit the heart. For example:

- In a study conducted among adults with diabetes, the patients drank 40 grams of concentrated pomegranate juice daily for eight weeks. The result was a significant reduction in total cholesterol, low-density lipoprotein (LDL) cholesterol, and the ratio of LDL and high-density lipoprotein (HDL) cholesterol. The researchers concluded that drinking pomegranate juice could improve heart disease risk factors in people who have high cholesterol.

- In a review published in the January 2009 issue of *Nutrition Review,* experts from Oklahoma State University noted that in previous studies, pomegranate juice had been shown to significantly reduce atherosclerotic lesions, systolic blood pressure in people with hypertension, and other indicators of heart health. They concluded that pomegranate juice has potential cardioprotective benefits and should be included in a heart-healthy diet.

- In a study of patients who had carotid artery stenosis, investigators asked them to consume pomegranate juice daily for either one or three years. Use of pomegranate juice reduced the size of arterial plaque by up to 30 percent while controls saw an increase of 9 percent during the first year of the study. Patients who drank the juice also had a significant improvement in systolic blood pressure.

The investigators concluded that these improvements could be associated with the potent polyphenols found in pomegranates.

RECIPE

We admit it: Eating a pomegranate can be a little messy and time-consuming. But because they are delicious, some people find it is well worth it. We won't ask you to tackle the fruit, however, so we offer an easy punch recipe.

Pomegranate Punch
Serves 1
1/2 cup pomegranate juice
1/2 cup fresh grapefruit juice
1/2 cup sparkling water

Combine all the ingredients and pour over ice.

RED WINE

Wine has been an honored and popular beverage for millennia. The earliest use of grapes to make wine is believed to have been about 9,000 years ago in China. The main ingredients, however, included rice, honey, and maybe grapes or Chinese hawthorn. Cultivation of grapes for wine is believed to have started by about 4000 B.C. and perhaps even 6000 B.C. Discovery of texts from tombs in Egypt show that wine was common around 2700 to 2500 B.C. The Old Testament mentions that Noah grew grapes and made wine.

In Europe, vineyards were managed under the control of the church and missions. In 1769, a Franciscan missionary named Father Junipero Serra platted the first

California vineyard at Mission San Diego. Father Serra went on to establish eight more vineyards and missions until he died in 1784.

Until the French chemist Louis Pasteur discovered that wine is made by microorganisms called yeasts, no one knew exactly how wine was produced. Pasteur's findings led to the discovery and development of different types of yeasts and eventually to better hygiene and better efficiency in wine production.

Types of red wine include cabernet sauvignon, chianti, merlot, sangiovese, and zinfandel. When it comes to nutritional value, all red wines are similar.

NUTRITIONAL VALUE—RED WINE
5 ounces red (generic)
Calories: 125
Potassium: 187 mg, 4% DRI

Why Red Wine Is Heart-Healthy

Don't let the lack of nutrients in the Nutritional Value table fool you: red wine gets its heart-healthy properties from phytonutrients, especially the flavonoids resveratrol and quercitin. Scientists have also identified other bioactive compounds, including monomeric and polymeric flavan-3-ols, anthocyanins, and phenolic acids, which likely also provide some benefits for the heart, although those benefits have yet to be determined.

Here's an interesting finding about resveratrol. Investigators who conducted a recent study (June 2009) of resveratrol suggest that up to 100 times more resveratrol is absorbed by the body if red wine is held in the mouth for a while (just how long was not mentioned), as the heart-healthy phytonutrient is mostly inactivated by the gut and liver before it reaches the blood.

Let's take a closer look at what some of the other studies say about red wine and heart disease.

- Quercitin and resveratrol appear to reduce the risk of heart disease by reducing platelet clumping and the formation of blood clots. They also protect against damage from LDL cholesterol.

- A Northwestern Ohio Universities College of Medicine study showed that resveratrol inhibits angiotensin II, a hormone that is secreted in response to high blood pressure and heart failure. Angiotensin II causes the secretion of collagen which results in stiffening of the heart muscle. Thus resveratrol prevents the damage angiotensin II can cause.

- The saponins found in the skin of grapes are believed to prevent the absorption of cholesterol and to reduce inflammation of blood vessels. Studies show that red wines contain 3 to 10 times the amount of saponins found in white wines.

- Resveratrol improves blood flow in the brain by 30 percent, according to a study published in the *Journal of Agricultural and Food Chemistry*. This greatly reduces the risk of stroke. The study's investigators hypothesized that resveratrol provides this advantage because it stimulates the production and/or release of nitric oxide, a substance manufactured in the lining of blood vessels that prompts the surrounding muscle to relax. This action expands the blood vessels and thus increases blood flow.

- A study published in the *American Journal of Clinical Nutrition* reports that in people who have high blood pressure, moderate consumption of red wine reduced the risk of death from coronary artery disease and other causes.

RECIPE

Sure, you can pour yourself a glass of red wine to have with dinner, but how about *eating* your wine? Here's a recipe that's a little different.

Red Wine Soup
Serves 4
4 cups vegetable broth
3 bay leaves
1/2 tsp dried thyme
3 cloves garlic, minced
2 Tbs olive oil
1 lb red onions, peeled and cut into thin slices
1/2 lb fresh tomatoes, peeled and chopped; or 1 cup canned whole tomatoes (save juice)
1/2 cup red wine
Salt and pepper to taste

Place the broth, bay leaves, and thyme in a pot, bring to a boil, and simmer for 20 minutes. Heat the oil in a big pot and add the onions. Cook on low heat for about 20–25 minutes. Stir often. While the onions are cooking, combine the minced garlic and tomatoes. (If using canned tomatoes, reserve the juice.) When the onions are soft, add the tomato mixture, 1 cup of broth, and salt to taste. Cover and cook for 15 minutes. Remove the cover and add the wine. Cook over medium heat until it reduces to about half. Pour in the remaining broth, bring to a boil, and simmer for 10 minutes. Add salt and pepper to taste.

SALMON

For people who eat fish, salmon is one of the most popular. There are two basic types of salmon sought by consumers: Atlantic and Pacific (including sockeye, Coho, Chinook, pink, and cherry).

One important question about salmon today is whether you should eat a farmed or wild fish. According to several studies, including one from Cornell University, farmed salmon have more omega-3 fatty acids (which are heart-healthy) than wild salmon, but the farmed fish also tend to have much higher levels of toxins that are known to cause cancer, neurobehavioral problems in children, and memory impairment.

Generally, one study showed that the net benefits of eating wild Pacific salmon outweighed those of eating farmed Atlantic salmon (most Atlantic salmon is farmed), although there are regional differences. Consumers also need to consider who is going to eat the fish. Individuals who have had a heart attack and who want to avoid having another one may benefit from eating farmed salmon. Pregnant women and young children, who can accumulate toxins in their bodies over time, should consider salmon that are least likely to contain harmful chemicals.

On average, farmed salmon contains two to three

times more beneficial fatty acids than wild salmon, apparently because of the diet they are fed. Chilean farmed salmon typically have very low levels of contaminants while European (especially Scottish) salmon show the highest levels. A study published in *Environmental Health Perspectives* (May 2005) found that contaminant levels are up to 10 times greater in farmed salmon than in wild Pacific salmon, and that European farmed salmon are more contaminated than salmon from South and North American farms.

NUTRITIONAL VALUE—ATLANTIC SALMON, FARMED
3 ounces, cooked, farmed
Calories: 175
Calcium: 13 mg
Niacin: 6.8 mg, 43% DRI
Potassium: 326 mg, 7% DRI
Selenium: 35 mg, 64% DRI
Thiamin: 0.3 mg, 25% DRI
Vitamin B_5: 1.3 mg, 26% DRI
Vitamin B_6: 0.5 mg, 29% DRI
Vitamin B_{12}: 2.38 mcg, 99% DRI

NUTRITIONAL VALUE—COHO, WILD
3 ounces, cooked
Calories: 118
Calcium: 38 mg
Niacin: 6.8 mg, 43% DRI
Potassium: 369 mg, 8% DRI
Selenium: 32 mg, 58% DRI
Vitamin B_5: 0.7 mg, 14% DRI
Vitamin B_6: 0.4 mg, 24% DRI
Vitamin B_{12}: 4.25 mcg, 177% DRI

NUTRITIONAL VALUE—SOCKEYE, WILD
3 ounces, cooked
Calories: 184
Niacin: 5.7 mg, 36% DRI
Potassium: 319 mg, 7% DRI
Vitamin B_5: 0.6 mg, 12% DRI
Vitamin B_{12}: 4.9 mcg, 204% DRI

Why Salmon Is Heart-Healthy

Omega-3 fatty acids and salmon seem to be synonymous: This fish is typically mentioned whenever people ask about foods that are rich in this heart-healthy nutrient. Salmon has some other heart-friendly components as well.

• The main omega-3 fatty acid found in salmon (EPA; eicosapentaenoic acid) is the immediate precursor of a type of prostaglandin that prevents platelets from sticking together and improves blood flow.

• Omega-3 fatty acids also improve the ratio of good to bad cholesterol, which ultimately helps prevent heart attack and stroke.

• A study published in the April 2005 issue of *Chest* reported that omega-3 fatty acids increase heart rate variability, which reduces the risk of arrhythmia and/or sudden death. In the study, researchers gave a 2-gram supplement of fish oil to half the elderly patients in the program for 11 weeks while the other half received soy oil. Patients in both groups had a significant increase in heart rate variability, but those who took the fish oil achieved a greater improvement in a shorter period of time. Those who took fish oil had a greater increase in heart rate variability within the first 2.7 weeks compared with 8.1 weeks in the placebo group.

• Salmon is also a good source of B vitamins. Niacin, for example, helps lower blood cholesterol, while B_{12} is necessary to reduce levels of the heart-damaging molecule called homocysteine.

• A study published in the *American Journal of Clinical Nutrition* (Chrysohoou) found that eating omega-3 rich fish improves the electrical properties of heart cells, which protects against deadly heart arrhythmias.

• You can reduce your risk of ischemic stroke by eating salmon just once a week, and significantly lower your risk if you eat it several times weekly. A study published in the January 17, 2006, issue of *Circulation* reported that people who ate omega-3-rich fish eight times per week had a 37 percent lower risk of developing coronary heart disease and a 56 percent lower risk of heart attack when compared with people who ate such fish once weekly.

• Scientists found that eating omega-3-rich fish such as salmon at least two times per week significantly reduces the progression of atherosclerosis among postmenopausal women. The study, which was published in the September

2004 issue of the *American Journal of Clinical Nutrition,* found that women who ate less than two servings of fish weekly had an average 4.54 percent increase in thickening and restriction in their arteries, while those who ate two servings weekly had an average increase of only 0.06 percent.

• People who consume greater amounts of omega-3 fatty acids have lower blood pressure than those who consume less, according to data collected in the International Study of Macro- and Micronutrients and Blood Pressure (INTERMAP) study. The average daily intake of omega-3 fatty acids was 2 grams. People who consumed more than 2 grams daily experienced a better reduction in blood pressure than those who ate less.

Overall, omega-3 fatty acids lower the amounts of cholesterol and triglycerides in the bloodstream, reduce platelet aggregation, help prevent thickening of the arteries, fight inflammation by reducing the production of chemicals called cytokines, and increase the activity of nitric oxide, which causes the arteries to relax.

RECIPE
This recipe is easy and quick. You may want to add your own special "twist" to the relish by adding chopped tomatoes, jalapeños, olives, or other ingredients. Enjoy!

Relished Salmon
Serves 4
Spray oil

4 salmon fillets, 6 oz each
2 cups water
6 Tbs chopped dill
1/4 cup wine vinegar
1 small onion, chopped
1/2 seedless cucumber, chopped
2 radishes, chopped
1 green bell pepper, seeded and chopped
Salt, pepper, and garlic powder to taste

Preheat oven to 400°F. Spray the bottom of a shallow baking dish with oil. Place the fillets in the dish and season with salt, pepper, and garlic powder. Add the water and 3 Tbs dill. Roast the fish for 12 to 15 minutes.

While the fish is cooking, combine the vinegar and chopped onions, cucumber, radishes, and pepper. Sprinkle in remaining 3 Tbs chopped dill and mix well. Remove the fish from the oven. Spoon pan juices over the fish and place fillets on dishes. Top fish with relish and serve.

SWEET POTATOES

These sweet root vegetables are among the oldest vegetables known. Sweet potatoes are native to Central America, where archaeologists have found proof in Peruvian caves that they were enjoyed as far back as 10,000 years ago.

Columbus brought sweet potatoes to Europe after his 1492 voyage to the New World. By the sixteenth century, Spanish explorers had brought the vegetable to the Philippines and the Portuguese had carried it to Africa, India, Indonesia, and southern Asia. About the same time, sweet potatoes were being cultivated in the southern U.S. The main producers of sweet potatoes today include China, Indonesia, Vietnam, Japan, India, and Uganda.

There are about 400 different varieties of sweet potato. The skin and flesh can range in color from nearly white to orange and pink and deep purple, although the most common types have white or yellow-orange flesh. The more intense the color of the flesh, the higher the beta-carotene content. Sweet potatoes that have purple flesh are rich in other phytonutrients—called anthocyanins—and in fact have the highest antioxidant properties of all sweet potato varieties.

Is it a yam or a sweet potato? The orange-colored vegetable most people call a yam is actually a sweet potato. A true yam belongs to the *Dioscoreae* family, while sweet potatoes belong to the *Convolvulaceae* or morning glory plant family.

NUTRITIONAL VALUE—SWEET POTATO
1 baked, medium (2" diameter, 5" long)
Calories: 103
Calcium: 43 mg
Fiber: 3.8 g, 12%
Iron: 0.8 mg, 10% DRI
Niacin: 1.7 mg, 10% DRI
Riboflavin: 0.12 mg, 9% DRI
Vitamin A: 21,909 IU, 730% DRI
Vitamin B_5: 1.0 mg, 20% DRI
Vitamin C: 22 mg, 24% DRI

Why Sweet Potatoes Are Heart-Healthy
Make sure you scrub your sweet potatoes well and eat the skin, because the skin has nearly three times more antioxidant activity than the rest of the vegetable.

- Sweet potatoes are an excellent source of beta-carotene and a very good source of vitamin C, both potent antioxidants. If you've heard that beta-carotene supplements may actually increase the risk of cardiovascular problems, be assured that the same is not true for *foods* that contain this nutrient. Studies show that people who eat foods rich in beta-carotene have a reduced risk of atherosclerosis, diabetic heart disease, and other heart-related conditions.

- The vitamin B_6 in sweet potatoes is necessary to help convert the heart-damaging amino acid called homocysteine into a benign substance.

- The potassium in sweet potatoes helps maintain fluid and electrolyte balance in the cells, as well as normal heart function and blood pressure. A recent review (August 2008) reported that reduced levels of potassium increases the risk of deadly ventricular arrhythmias in people who have ischemic heart disease, heart failure, and left ventricular hypertrophy. An increased intake of potassium can help prevent this, and the best way to increase potassium intake is to eat more foods rich in potassium, like sweet potatoes.

RECIPE
This may be the easiest sweet potato recipe ever. All you need is a grill—and if you don't have one, use a skillet. It won't be exactly the same, but close.

Grilled Sweet Potatoes
4 sweet potatoes, scrubbed
BBQ sauce or your favorite grilling sauce

*Cut each sweet potato lengthwise into "steaklike" pieces,
each about ¼ inch thick. Brush each piece on both sides
with your favorite sauce. Place on a hot grill or skillet.
Cook until tender and brown.*

TEMPEH

Tempeh is not a household word—nor a common menu
item—in the United States, but this highly nutritious food
with its unique taste and texture is gaining popularity in
America. The fermented soybean food has been a staple
in the diet of people in Indonesia for more than two millennia. The Dutch introduced tempeh to Europe after they
colonized Indonesia, but the soy-based food did not make
its way to the United States until the twentieth century.

Tempeh is made by cooking and dehulling soybeans,
treating them with a culturing agent, and then allowing
them to ferment until the result is a solid cake. The texture is sometimes described as being nougat-like and the
taste as being nutty, although tempeh tends to absorb the
flavors of the foods and sauces with which it is prepared.
Regular tempeh is typically made from soybeans, rice,
and tempeh culture, but some tempeh products also
contain grains such as brown rice, oats, millet, and/or
barley.

NUTRITIONAL VALUE—TEMPEH
3.5 ounces
Calories: 196

Fiber: 7 g, 22%
Calcium: 96 mg
Iron: 2.1 mg, 26% DRI
Magnesium: 77 mg, 18% DRI
Niacin: 2.1 mg, 13% DRI
Potassium: 401 mg, 9% DRI

Why Tempeh Is Heart-Healthy

Tempeh offers high levels of several vitamins and minerals, as well as an excellent amount of protein while contributing much less saturated fat than animal sources of protein. Unlike animal proteins, tempeh does not have any cholesterol, which makes it a heart-healthy alternative to animal protein any day!

- The soy protein in tempeh tends to reduce cholesterol levels. In a meta-analysis of 41 randomized controlled trials in which soy protein was the only substance evaluated, soy protein was associated with a significant reduction in total cholesterol (mean, 5.2 mg/dL), low-density lipoprotein (LDL) (mean, 4.2 mg/dL), and triglycerides (mean, 6.2 mg/dL). Soy protein also significantly raised "good" HDL cholesterol levels (mean, 0.77 mg/dL).

- Magnesium is in good supply in tempeh, and this mineral is known for its ability to relax blood vessels. This puts it in the plus column as benefiting the cardiovascular system.

- The fiber in tempeh binds to cholesterol and fats and helps remove them from the body, which lowers cholesterol levels.

RECIPE

Tempeh may not have been on your menu before, but once you try it, chances are pretty good you'll be back for more. High in protein and very versatile, tempeh is a tasty alternative to animal protein. Enjoy!

Lemon Broiled Tempeh
2 8-oz packs of any style tempeh
1 medium onion, sliced into rings
1 cup mushrooms
1/3 cup lemon juice, fresh
1/8 cup olive oil
1/4 cup soy sauce
4 cloves of garlic, minced

Cut the tempeh into 2" squares. Arrange them in a glass 9"×13" baking pan. In a small bowl, mix the lemon juice, olive oil, soy sauce, and garlic. Place the onion rings and mushrooms on top of the tempeh squares and pour the lemon juice mixture over them. Allow the tempeh to marinate for 4 to 6 hours, basting occasionally. Bake at 400° for 25 minutes. During the final 5 minutes, turn the tempeh and broil for 5 minutes.

TOFU

Tofu was discovered more than 2,000 years ago, most likely by serendipity, in China. This high-protein and nutritious food is frequently called "the cheese of Asia" because it looks like a block of farmer's cheese. Tofu is made from the curds of soybean milk and is a staple food in most Asian countries.

Tofu was introduced to the Japanese in the eighth

century, but it did not become widely popular there until the seventeenth century. Tofu's popularity in the West didn't gain momentum until the 1960s, when it was recognized as a health food and for its versatility. Because tofu has a neutral taste and readily absorbs the flavors of other ingredients, it can be used in a wide variety of recipes, ranging from desserts to entrées. It is also available in several consistencies, including silken, soft, firm, and extra firm.

NUTRITIONAL VALUE—TOFU, EXTRA FIRM
Approx. 3 ounces, Vitasoy extra firm
Calories: 77
Fiber: 1 g, 3%
Calcium: 61 mg
Iron: 1.26 mg, 16% DRI

NUTRITIONAL VALUE—TOFU, SILKEN/SOFT
3 ounces, Mori-Nu
Calories: 46
Fiber: 0.1 g, 0%
Calcium: 26 mg
Potassium: 151 mg, 3% DRI

Why Tofu Is Heart-Healthy

You have likely heard some debate and controversy over the health benefits of tofu and soy protein. As with nearly everything in life, moderation is the key. The heart-healthy advantages provided by tofu and soy protein are clear in many different studies, a few of which we present here.

- Just 4 ounces of tofu provides 14.4 percent of the daily value for omega-3 fatty acids, which help prevent arrhythmia and make the blood less likely to clot and block the arteries. Omega-3 fatty acids also improve the ratio of good HDL to bad LDL cholesterol.

• A meta-analysis of eleven studies was done to evaluate the effects of soy isoflavones (phytonutrients in soybeans/tofu) on lipid (cholesterol, triglyceride) levels. The investigators found that soy isoflavones significantly decreased total cholesterol and LDL cholesterol levels, and significantly increased HDL cholesterol. The reductions in LDL cholesterol were greater in people who have high cholesterol than in those who had normal cholesterol.

• In another meta-analysis, this time of 41 randomized controlled trials, the investigators found that soy protein supplementation reduced total cholesterol, LDL cholesterol, and triglycerides, and also increased HDL cholesterol. They concluded that replacing foods high in saturated fat and cholesterol with soy protein foods (e.g., tofu, tempeh) may be beneficial when it comes to coronary risk factors.

It is worth noting that in 1999, the Food and Drug Administration (FDA) approved soy protein's health claim, namely that the daily consumption of 25 grams of soy reduces the risk of heart disease and lowers cholesterol levels.

RECIPE

Here is an alternative to the traditional beef burger. These tofu burgers can be enjoyed on whole wheat buns with all the regular toppings—tomatoes, lettuce, onions, and ketchup. These burgers taste especially great on the grill.

Tofu Burgers
Makes 4–6
1 lb extra firm tofu
1/4 cup each whole wheat flour, corn flour, and rolled oats
1 Tbs minced garlic
1/2 cup parsley or fresh basil leaves, dried
1 tsp each paprika, coriander, cumin
1/2 tsp dried basil or thyme
1 Tbs soy sauce

Heat a nonstick frying pan using spray cooking oil and add the minced garlic and sauté it. Cut the tofu into 1-inch chunks and put in a food processor or mash by hand. Finely chop the basil. Place all of the ingredients into the processor or bowl and mix well. Form the mixture into thin patties and fry (using extra spray oil as needed) on medium heat for 5 to 7 minutes on each side or until brown.

TOMATOES

Few things say "summer fresh" better than a sun-ripened tomato on the vine. Be they red, yellow, or orange or the less common purple or brown, tomatoes are delicious and loaded with phytonutrients.

Although you find tomatoes in the vegetable aisle,

they are really fruits. The original tomatoes, which were natives of the western side of South America, were probably about the size of grape or cherry tomatoes. The Mexicans were the first culture to cultivate tomatoes, and when the Spanish conquistadors entered Mexico, they were introduced to the fruit and brought the seeds back to Spain.

It may be hard to believe that when tomatoes got to Italy, the Italians believed they were poisonous because the plant is a member of the deadly nightshade family. They were half right: the leaves but not the fruits contain toxic alkaloids. It was several centuries before Italians embraced tomatoes—and thus sauce!

In North America, tomatoes are believed to have been first introduced in Massachusetts, but they did not become popular until the late nineteenth century. Today, however, they are among the most popular "vegetables" in the United States. Top producers of tomatoes include the United States, Russia, Italy, Spain, China, and Turkey.

NUTRITIONAL VALUE—TOMATO
1 large (3" diameter), raw
Calories: 33
Fiber: 2.2 g, 7%
Iron: 0.5 mg, 6% DRI
Potassium: 431 mg, 9% DRI
Vitamin A: 1,516 IU, 51% DRI
Vitamin C: 23 mg, 26% DRI

Why Tomatoes Are Heart-Healthy
Although tomatoes are a powerhouse of nutrients, they may be best known for their high content of lycopene, a

potent phytonutrient and antioxidant associated with fighting cancer. Lycopene also provides cardiovascular benefits, as do several other nutrients found in this luscious fruit. Here's what the studies say.

- A study conducted at Brigham and Women's Hospital in Boston, Massachusetts, found that consuming lots of lycopene-rich foods can reduce the risk of cardiovascular disease. Nearly 40,000 women middle-aged and older were studied, and during more than seven years of follow-up, those who ate seven to 10 servings of lycopene-rich foods per week had a 29 percent lower risk of cardiovascular disease when compared to women who consumed less than 1.5 servings weekly. Women who ate more than two servings per week of oil-based tomato foods (e.g., tomato sauce, pizza) had a 34 percent lower risk.

- Tomatoes are a very good source of potassium, a nutrient that helps reduce high blood pressure and thus the risk of heart disease.

- Niacin is known to safely lower high cholesterol levels, and tomatoes are a good source of this B vitamin.

- The combination of vitamin B_6 and folic acid in tomatoes team up to transform homocysteine into harmless molecules. High levels of homocysteine damage blood vessels and increase the risk of stroke and heart attack.

- A European study published in the *European Journal of Nutrition* found that women who ate tomato products that provided them with 8 mg of lycopene daily for three weeks were much less likely to experience plaque formation associated with LDL cholesterol.

- The value of lycopene in preventing heart disease continues to be impressive. In a 4.8-year study published in the *Journal of Nutrition*, investigators found that women who consumed the most lycopene-rich, tomato-based foods had the lowest risk for cardiovascular disease. Overall, women whose blood lycopene levels were the highest had a 50 percent reduced risk of cardiovascular disease compared to women who had the lowest blood levels.

- An Australian study published in the *Journal of the American Medical Association* found that among people who had type 2 diabetes, those who consumed 8 ounces of tomato juice daily had significantly reduced clumping of platelets than diabetics who took placebo. Because clumping platelets stick to the lining of blood vessel walls, they can lead to the development of cardiovascular disease.

RECIPE

Hands down, the best tomato recipe for providing excellent amounts of heart-healthy nutrients is gazpacho. Easy to make (except for the chopping) and requires no cooking. Make it as spicy as you like and enjoy it any time.

Gazpacho
Serves 4
4 cups tomato or vegetable cocktail juice (spicy or not)
1 large cucumber, peeled and chopped fine
4 medium tomatoes, chopped fine
2 stalks celery, chopped fine
1 yellow bell pepper, seeded and chopped fine
1 green bell pepper, seeded and chopped fine
2 cloves garlic, minced
1/4 cup red wine vinegar
1 tsp lemon juice
Several dashes of hot sauce (optional)

Combine all ingredients in a large pot or serving bowl, chill for about 1 hour, and serve.

TUNA

According to the National Fisheries Institute, canned tuna is the second most popular and most consumed fish in the United States, narrowly beating out salmon and topped only by shrimp. Tuna's popularity is a good thing, because of its heart-healthy properties. But more about that later.

People have been enjoying tuna ever since they could catch them. The flesh is dense and has a meaty texture. Ancient people typically pickled and smoked tuna, which allowed them to prevent it from spoiling quickly.

Tuna is fished in warm water in the Pacific, Atlantic, and Indian oceans, and in the Mediterranean Sea. Several varieties include bluefish and yellowfin, which have red flesh, and albacore, which is pink.

One concern surrounding tuna is mercury contamination. The Food and Drug Administration (FDA) advises consumers on the risks of eating fish and shellfish, especially young children and women of childbearing age. Generally the FDA makes the following recommendations for eating fish and shellfish (including tuna), and notes that young children should be given small amounts.

- Eat up to 12 ounces per week of fish lower in mercury, which includes canned light tuna, shrimp, salmon, pollack, and catfish.

- Albacore ("white") tuna contains more mercury than canned light tuna. Thus you should not consume more than 6 ounces of albacore tuna weekly.

NUTRITIONAL VALUE—TUNA, LIGHT
Canned, in water, drained, 3 oz
Calories: 99
Iron: 1.3 mg, 16% DRI
Niacin: 11.3 mg, 71% DRI
Selenium: 68 mg, 123% DRI
Vitamin B_6: 0.3 mg, 18% DRI
Vitamin B_{12}: 2.54 mcg, 106% DRI

NUTRITIONAL VALUE—TUNA, FRESH YELLOWFIN
Cooked, 3 oz
Calories: 118
Fiber: 0 g
Iron: 0.8 mg, 10% DRI
Niacin: 10.1 mg, 63% DRI

Selenium: 40 mg, 73% DRI
Vitamin B$_5$: 0.7 mg, 14% DRI
Vitamin B$_6$: 0.9 mg, 53% DRI
Vitamin B$_{12}$: 0.5 mcg, 21% DRI

Why Tuna Is Heart-Healthy

Like salmon, tuna is an excellent source of omega-3 fatty acids, so there are many heart benefits that go along with them. Tuna is also a great source of vitamin B$_{12}$, niacin, selenium, and vitamin B$_6$. The studies have this to say about the goodness of tuna.

- The omega-3 fatty acids in tuna increase heart rate variability, which reduces the risk of sudden death and/or arrhythmia. A study published in the April 2005 issue of *Chest* found that after only 2.7 weeks of taking 2 grams of fish oil daily, patients experienced a significant increase in heart rate variability, compared with 8.1 weeks for patients who took soy oil.

- Eating tuna can lower your triglyceride levels, which reduces your risk of cardiovascular disease. In a six-month study that included 142 overweight adults who had high triglyceride levels, those who consumed two servings of fish high in omega-3s plus used canola oil had a 10.4 percent decline in triglyceride levels.

- Eating tuna can also help reduce the risk of certain types of stroke. A 15-year study that involved nearly 80,000 women found that those who ate fish 2 to 4 times weekly had a 27 percent reduced risk of stroke compared to women who ate fish only once a month. Those who ate fish five or more times weekly reduce their risk of certain stroke by 52 percent.

- Tuna also protects against heart attack. A study published in the January 17, 2006, issue of *Circulation* followed 41,578 adults aged 40 to 59. The investigators found that the risk of coronary heart disease was reduced by 42 percent among the participants who ate 2.1 grams daily of omega-3 fatty acids compared to those who ate only 300 milligrams daily.

- Tuna is an excellent source of selenium, a mineral and antioxidant that has been shown in some studies to provide protection against oxidative stress in myocardial ischemia.

- Both vitamin B_{12} and vitamin B_6 are found in good amounts in tuna, and these vitamins are essential for lowering levels of homocysteine, a compound that is an important risk factor for atherosclerosis.

RECIPE

Although canned tuna is very popular, we decided to offer a fresh tuna recipe. If you have never tried fresh tuna, we hope you give this one a try. It's easy, quick, and delicious!

Spicy Tuna
Serves 4
2 lb tuna steaks

⅛ cup olive oil
4 cloves garlic, minced
2 Tbs soy sauce
¼ tsp dry mustard
½ tsp black pepper
3 Tbs fresh lemon juice
1 lemon, cut in wedges

In a jar, combine the oil, garlic, soy sauce, mustard, lemon juice, and pepper. Shake well. Rinse the tuna steaks and pat dry. Place the tuna in a shallow pan and pour the marinade over them. Cover the pan and refrigerate the tuna for 1 hour. Cook the tuna on a lightly oiled broiler pan for 4 to 5 minutes on each side or until the tuna is opaque. Serve with lemon wedges.

WALNUTS

Some say the kernel of the walnut looks like a brain; a more aesthetic perspective is that the two lobes look like a butterfly. Regardless of how you see a walnut, you will be looking at a popular tree nut that has been cultivated for thousands of years. And depending on the type of walnut, the place of origin changes.

The English (or Persian) walnut, which is the most popular type in the United States, originated in India. The ancient Romans introduced this walnut to the European countries. When the English sailed to the New World, they brought the walnuts with them, and hence the name.

Although English walnuts are American favorites, its two cousins—black walnuts and white walnuts—are both native to North America. Their less popular status may be due to a few factors: black walnuts have thicker shells than the English variety and thus are much harder to crack. White walnuts, although sweeter than their cousins, are also oilier and the least common.

The United States, as well as Turkey, China, Iran, France, and Romania, are the main producers of walnuts.

NUTRITIONAL VALUE—WALNUTS
1 ounce, English walnuts
Calories: 185
Fiber: 1.9 g, 6%
Calcium: 28 mg
Iron: 0.8 mg, 10% DRI

Why Walnuts Are Heart-Healthy
Who says walnuts are good for your heart? Well, the Food and Drug Administration (FDA), for one. The FDA has stated, "Eating 1.5 ounces per day of walnuts as part of a diet low in saturated fat and cholesterol may reduce the risk of heart disease." What are the study results that led the FDA to make this claim? Here are a few.

- The *Journal of Nutrition* published a study in which 23 adults who had elevated LDL cholesterol levels were assigned to one of three diets on a rotating six-week basis with a two-week break between each one. Diet 1 was the standard American diet; diet 2 was a linoleic acid diet that included one ounce of walnuts and a teaspoon of walnut oil daily; diet 3 was an alpha-linoleic acid diet that added one teaspoon of flaxseed oil to

diet two. Both diets 2 and 3 reduced LDL cholesterol levels, lowered levels of C-reactive protein
(a marker of inflammation associated with heart
disease), decreased levels of substances called
ICAM-1, VCAM-1, and E-selection, which help
cholesterol stick to the lining of arteries, and increased levels of omega-3 fatty acids.

- Walnuts are an excellent source of monounsaturated fats, which help reduce LDL and total cholesterol levels, as well as levels of Lp(a), a lipid
that is a risk factor for atherosclerosis when elevated.

- Walnuts have high levels of the essential amino
acid I-arginine, which plays a role in reducing
hypertension. L-arginine converts into nitric
oxide, a chemical that allows blood vessels to
relax and helps keep the inside of blood vessels
smooth.

- The omega-3 fatty acids in walnuts help the cardiovascular system by reducing the tendency
for blood to clot inside arteries, improving the
ratio of good (HDL) cholesterol to bad (LDL)
cholesterol, and reducing inflammation, which
is a key factor in causing cholesterol to form
plaque.

- An article in *Phytochemistry* states that polyphenolic compounds called ellagic and gallic acid,
which are found in walnuts, have the ability to inhibit the free radical damage to LDL cholesterol.

But that's not all: the researchers named a total of 16 polyphenols that have "remarkable" antioxidant properties.

- A review published in the *British Journal of Nutrition* evaluated four large epidemiological studies. When all the data were combined, the results showed that people who ate nuts at least four times a week had a 37 percent reduced risk of coronary heart disease compared to those who never or seldom ate nuts. For each additional serving of nuts individuals ate per week, they could enjoy an additional 8.3 percent reduction in their risk of coronary heart disease.

RECIPE

Walnuts are great all by themselves, fresh out of the shell, sprinkled on cereal or yogurt, or in a trail mix. But we want to offer you a recipe that is a little different.

Zucchini and Walnuts
Serves 4
1/2 cup walnuts, coarsely chopped
1 1/2 lbs zucchini
Salt and black pepper to taste
1 clove garlic, minced
2 Tbs olive oil

In a large skillet, heat 1 Tbs oil and toss in the walnuts and garlic. Stir until the nuts are lightly brown (about 8 minutes), then remove from the pan. Trim the ends from the zucchini and slice into 1/2 inch thick slices. Heat 1 Tbs olive oil in the pan and sauté the zucchini until they begin to get soft. Combine the walnut mixture with the zucchini in a serving dish and season with salt and pepper. Serve.

WHEAT GERM

Wheat germ is the embryo of wheat, the nutrient dense portion of the wheat kernel. The term "germ" refers to germination. Although the germ makes up only about 2 percent of the wheat kernel, it contains the most nutrients in the kernel. In fact, wheat germ contains 23 nutrients, more per ounce than any other grain or vegetable. The germ is the part of the wheat that is removed during the process of converting whole wheat flour to white flour.

NUTRITIONAL VALUE—WHEAT GERM, PLAIN, TOASTED

2 ounces
Calories: 217
Fiber: 8.6 g, 27%
Calcium: 26 mg
Folic acid: 200 mcg, 50% DRI
Iron: 5 mg, 62% DRI
Manganese: 11.3 mg, 491% DRI
Niacin: 3.1 mg, 19% DRI
Potassium: 537 mg, 11% DRI
Riboflavin: 0.5 mg, 38% DRI
Selenium: 37 mg, 67% DRI
Thiamin: 0.95 mg, 79% DRI
Vitamin B_6: 0.6 mg, 35% DRI
Zinc: 9.5 mg, 86% DRI

Why Wheat Germ Is Heart-Healthy

As the nutritional value chart shows, wheat germ contains a wealth of nutrients. It also contains octacosanol, a waxy substance found in some plant oils. Wheat germ is one of the few foods that contain high levels of this molecule. Various studies show how some of these nutrients can benefit the heart.

- In a recent animal study done in France, the researchers fed wheat germ to rats and found that it very effectively decreased the susceptibility of heart and liver lipids (cholesterols, triglycerides) to oxidation. This is important, as oxidation is a process that damages the heart and heart function.

- There is some evidence that octacosanol can reduce cholesterol. A 2006 Spanish study reports that octacosanol is among a group of plant elements called stanols and sterols that reduce absorption of cholesterol by the intestinal tract and decrease total and LDL cholesterol by about 10 percent. A University of Georgia study also indicates that octacosanol may reduce LDL and increase HDL cholesterol levels. Further research is needed.

- Wheat germ is very high in fiber, which is important in helping reduce cholesterol in the blood and thus reduce the risk of atherosclerosis and heart disease.

- Just 2 ounces of wheat germ provides 50 percent of the daily requirement for folic acid, a B vitamin that is critical for helping reduce levels of heart-damaging homocysteine.

- Wheat germ is a very rich source of manganese. A manganese deficiency is associated with high blood pressure, high cholesterol, and various heart conditions. Although manganese deficiency is not common, low levels occur in some people, as significant amounts of manganese are lost during food processing.

- An animal study has indicated that zinc may help prevent atherosclerosis. The results showed that although the mineral did not affect the amount of cholesterol in the blood, it had a significant impact on removing cholesterol that had accumulated on the artery walls.

RECIPE
The most common way to enjoy wheat germ is to sprinkle it on cereal, although many also enjoy it on ice cream, pudding, fruit salads, and vegetables. While we encourage you to use wheat germ in these ways, you may also find the following recipe to be a delightful change of pace.

What's Shaking Shake
Serves 1
1 cup plain no-fat yogurt
1/2 cup nonfat milk or soymilk
1 ripe banana

3 walnuts
3 Tbs wheat germ

Place all ingredients in a food processor or blender and process until smooth.

WINTER SQUASH

Winter squash are members of the *Cucurbitaceae* family and relatives of cucumber and melon. Although there are many different varieties with various colors, flavors, sizes, and shapes, they all share several characteristics. All have hard shells, which allows them to be stored for as long as six months. Each variety also has a hollow inner core that harbors seeds, and the flesh is typically mildly sweet and somewhat grained.

Modern-day winter squash originated in the region bordering Mexico and Guatemala, where people have been eating different varieties for more than 10,000 years. Unlike the winter squash you find in markets today, the first cultivated varieties contained mostly seeds, and these rather than the flesh were what the people ate, as the flesh had a bitter taste.

Over time, squash was cultivated throughout the Americas, and a sweet-tasting flesh developed. Columbus is credited with bringing squash to Europe, and from there the Spanish and Portuguese explorers carried it throughout the world. Today most squash is grown in China, Japan, Romania, Turkey, Italy, Egypt, and Argentina.

Here are some of the more common winter squash varieties:

- Butternut squash: Shaped like a large pear, this squash has cream-colored skin, deep orange-colored flesh and a sweet flavor.

- Acorn squash: With harvest green skin speckled with orange patches and pale yellow-orange flesh, this squash has a unique flavor that is a combination of sweet, nutty and peppery.

- Hubbard squash: A larger-sized squash that can be dark green, gray-blue or orange-red in color, the Hubbard's flavor is less sweet than many other varieties.

- Spaghetti squash: A spaghetti squash averages from 4 to 8 pounds and is cylinder-shaped. A true spaghetti squash is pale ivory to pale yellow, although an orange variety was developed in the early 1990s, which is higher in beta-carotene than its paler cousins.

- Turban squash: Green in color and either speckled or striped, this winter squash has an orange-yellow flesh whose taste is reminiscent of hazelnuts.

- Pumpkins: The pumpkin with the most flesh and sweetest taste is the small-sized one known as sugar or pie pumpkin, the latter referring to its most notable culinary usage.

NUTRITIONAL VALUE—ACORN SQUASH
1 cup, cubed, baked
Calories: 115
Fiber: 9 g, 28%
Calcium: 90 mg
Iron: 1.9 mg, 23% DRI
Potassium: 896 mg, 19% DRI
Vitamin C: 22 mg, 24% DRI

NUTRITIONAL VALUE—SPAGHETTI SQUASH
1 cup
Calories: 42
Fiber: 2.2 g, 7%
Calcium: 33 mg
Iron: 0.5 mg, 6% DRI
Niacin: 1.3 mg, 8% DRI
Potassium: 181 mg, 4% DRI
Vitamin A: 170 IU, 6% DRI

Why Winter Squash Are Heart-Healthy
Winter squash, unlike their cousins that grow in the summer (e.g., yellow squash, zucchini), can be gathered very late into the autumn and be stored for months and still retain their nutritional and heart-friendly value. Let's look at what the research says about the virtues of winter squash.

- In a recent Italian study, investigators noted that low plasma concentrations of antioxidant vitamins (beta-carotene, A, and E) were associated with carotid atherosclerosis, and that regular intake of foods rich in these antioxidants may slow progression of the disease. Winter squash are an excellent source of vitamin A/beta-carotene.

- Folic acid is critical for reducing heart-damaging homocysteine levels, and winter squash is a good source of this nutrient.

- Beta-carotene is both an antioxidant and anti-inflammatory, and winter squash is an excellent source. These properties enable winter squash to help prevent the oxidation of cholesterol, which is critical because oxidized cholesterol is the type that accumulates in blood vessels and can lead to stroke and heart attack.

- Fiber is necessary to help eliminate artery-clogging cholesterol, and winter squash is a good source.

- Winter squash is rich in carotenoids that can help regulate blood sugar levels. This is especially important for people at risk for heart disease, as insulin resistance and high blood sugar levels are part of the metabolic syndrome, a known risk factor for heart disease.

RECIPE

With such a wide variety of winter squash to choose from, it was hard to pick one. So we chose a recipe in which you could substitute any of the squash. Feel free to select your favorite, or choose several.

Middle Eastern Squash

Serves 8
4 lb of your favorite winter squash
3 Tbs olive oil
1/2 tsp ground cardamom

³/₄ tsp ground coriander
¹/₈ tsp ground ginger
¹/₈ tsp allspice
¹/₂ cup toasted slivered almonds
Zest of 1 orange
Salt and pepper to taste

Cook the squash of your choice until tender and cut into one-inch chunks. In a large skillet, heat the oil and all the spices (except the salt and pepper) over medium heat for about 1 minute. Stir in the cooked squash and sauté until well coated. Add salt and pepper to taste. Sprinkle with toasted almonds and orange zest just before you serve.

YOGURT

Yogurt (from the Turkish name "yoghurmak," which means "to thicken") is a fermented dairy food that is made by adding bacterial cultures to milk. These "good" or beneficial bacteria transform the sugar (lactose) in the milk into lactic acid, the substance that gives yogurt its unique taste and texture.

Experts are not sure when or where yogurt was first made, although fermented dairy foods have been a regular part of the diet of many cultures ever since cows were domesticated. There is a record of yogurt being consumed during the thirteenth century in the Middle East, which is just one of the places where this pudding-like food has been and continues to be a favorite. Other places where yogurt is a major part of the cuisine include Turkey, Greece, India, Eastern Europe, and Asia.

The health benefits of yogurt were not explored scientifically until the twentieth century, when Dr. Elie Metchnikoff studied the lactic-acid-producing bacteria in the fermented dairy product and found an association between eating yogurt and longevity in certain cultures, such as the Bulgarians, who eat a lot of yogurt. The heart-related benefits have been discovered more recently.

NUTRITIONAL VALUE—YOGURT, PLAIN, LOW-FAT
8 ounces
Calories: 154
Calcium: 448 mg
Potassium: 573 mg, 12% DRI
Riboflavin: 0.5 mg, 38% DRI
Thiamin: 0.1 mg, 8% DRI
Vitamin B_6: 0.12 mg, 7% DRI
Vitamin B_{12}: 1.37 mcg, 57% DRI

Why Yogurt Is Heart-Healthy

Low-fat dairy foods are a good source of calcium, protein, B-complex vitamins, potassium, magnesium, and other important nutrients that are good for the heart. Yogurt is an especially nutritious choice because it also contains beneficial bacteria (probiotics), which can support the immune system and fight off infections, improve digestion, and enhance absorption of nutrients, which can directly benefit heart function. Here are a few studies that highlight the heart-healthy benefits of yogurt.

- A review conducted by Washington State University reported on the results from several studies which showed that intake of dairy foods reduces the risk of stroke and reduces blood pressure. The review's author notes that three minerals—

calcium, magnesium, and potassium—appear to contribute to the reduction in blood pressure and stroke, and that yogurt is an especially good source of these minerals.

• A study published in the *Annals of Nutrition & Metabolism* reports that yogurt can significantly improve cholesterol levels. During the six-week study, one group of women consumed 3 ounces of probiotic yogurt daily for two weeks, while a second group of 16 women ate yogurt without probiotics for two weeks. For the next two weeks, both groups of women increased their daily intake to 6 ounces. During the final two weeks, none of the women ate yogurt. When the women's cholesterol levels were checked, the researchers found that the women who had consumed the probiotic yogurt experienced a significant decline in their LDL (bad) cholesterol and a substantial increase in their good (HDL) cholesterol levels. The women who had eaten the nonprobiotic yogurt also had a significant decline in LDL cholesterol, but their HDL levels did not rise.

• In the Rotterdam Study, researchers were looking for a relationship between intake of dairy foods and hypertension. The study included 2,245 participants age 55 years or older who did not have high blood pressure when the study began. The dairy food intake and blood pressure of the subjects were followed for six years. At the six-year follow-up, the researchers analyzed their data and concluded that intake of low-fat dairy products may contribute to the prevention of hypertension in older adults.

CHAPTER 5

Heart-Healthy Supplements: A to Z

Scientists have found a number of natural supplements that are easy to use and that can promote a healthy heart and cardiovascular system. In this chapter we explore 12 of those supplements, providing you with a description of the item, the properties that make it a heart-healthy candidate, the science behind the claims, any precautions for use, and the typical dose. These supplements often can be taken along with conventional medications for the prevention and treatment of heart disease. However, we strongly encourage you to talk to your health-care provider before starting any supplement program.

CARNITINE

Carnitine (often referred to as L-carnitine) is an amino acid that is formed from two others—lysine and methionine. It is produced by the body in the liver and kidneys and stored in the heart, brain, skeletal muscles, and sperm.

Along with being an antioxidant and fighting free

radicals, carnitine also plays a role in energy production because it transfers omega-3 fatty acids into the mitochondria, which is the energy-producing factory in the body's cells. Carnitine is essential for transforming fat into energy.

Although the body can usually produce all the carnitine it needs, some people may have a deficiency or be unable to transport it efficiently to their cells. Heart-related conditions such as angina or intermittent claudication (severe, cramp-like pain that occurs in the legs during exercise) can cause insufficient levels of carnitine, as can use of some medications such as valproic acid and its derivatives.

Why Carnitine Is Heart-Healthy

The heart gets about 60 percent of its fuel from fat; carnitine is important for heart health because it plays a critical role in changing fat into energy. Because carnitine also enhances the metabolism of fatty acids, it also prevents the accumulation of toxic fat metabolites. These factors and more make carnitine a heart-healthy supplement.

- In a study published in January 2009, 81 people who had type 2 diabetes were randomly assigned to receive either 2 grams carnitine or placebo daily for three months. After three months, the patients who had taken carnitine had significant improvement in their levels of oxidized low-density lipoprotein (LDL) cholesterol compared with the placebo group. This is critical, because oxidized LDL damages blood vessels and thus the heart. Patients in the carnitine group also had a significant decline in their triglyceride levels and an improvement in oxidative stress.

• Several clinical trials have shown that carnitine can help reduce symptoms of angina.

• A few small studies suggest that people who take carnitine after they have suffered a heart attack may be less likely to experience a subsequent attack, die of heart disease, or develop heart failure. The carnitine in such cases was taken along with conventional medications.

• There is some evidence that carnitine can help reduce symptoms of peripheral vascular disease and help individuals who have intermittent claudication walk a greater distance.

How to Take Carnitine

The suggested doses of carnitine depend on what condition you are treating. For example, if you have angina or heart failure, a recommended dose is 1.5 to 2 grams daily. People with heart disease may be prescribed 600 to 1,200 mg three times daily, or 750 mg twice daily. A recommended dose for peripheral artery disease is 2 to 4 grams daily.

Side effects, which rarely occur, are usually mild. If you take 5 or more grams per day you may experience diarrhea. Other side effects may include body odor, rash, and increased appetite.

Although you should always consult your doctor before starting any supplement program, it is especially important to talk to your physician before taking carnitine if you have any of the following conditions: hypertension, cirrhosis, diabetes, kidney disease, or peripheral vascular disease.

CAYENNE

Cayenne, or cayenne pepper *(Capsicum frutescens)*, is an herb and herbal supplement made from the dried pods of chili peppers that grow on the plant. The shrubby perennial, which can grow up to six feet high, originated in Central and South America, where it has been cultivated for more than seven thousand years. The word *cayenne* comes from the Greek "to bite," which is in reference to the hot pungent properties of the peppers and the seeds.

Cayenne has been used for medicinal purposes for millennia. The main healing properties of cayenne come from a chemical called capsaicin, which is the substance that gives the peppers their heat. Generally, the more the pepper burns your mouth, the more capsaicin it contains.

Why Cayenne Is Heart-Healthy

People around the world use cayenne to treat various health problems, including poor circulation, heart disease, and many nonheart-related conditions. Here we focus on the heart-related benefits.

- Cayenne has the ability to prevent platelets from sticking together and forming blood clots, while also increasing the body's ability to dissolve fibrin, a substance that is involved in the formation of blood clots. This makes the herb helpful in preventing stroke and heart attack.

- An Australian study looked at the impact of cayenne chili on vascular function and the heart in healthy men. They found that cayenne improved resting heart rate and increased effective myocardial perfusion pressure time.

- Although several animal studies have shown that cayenne effectively reduces blood cholesterol and triglyceride levels, there are few studies in humans. One done in Australia showed that healthy adults who regularly consumed cayenne chili for four weeks had a significantly lower oxidation rate than people who did not consume cayenne. A lower oxidation rate is important, as it protects against heart damage.

- Other studies show that cayenne increases and improves blood circulation, which can be especially helpful for people who are at risk for or who have peripheral artery disease.

How to Take Cayenne

Cayenne is available in capsules and as a powder. Some experts recommend taking the powder because its healing powers can begin right away. If you put cayenne into your mouth, your stomach detects it and begins to secrete digestive juices and thus prepares the stomach for when the cayenne arrives. It also stimulates the nerve endings and immediately sends signals throughout the body, which in turn sends blood flowing right away. If you take a capsule, the cayenne is released into the stomach without warning, the body does not respond immediately, and increased blood flow is delayed.

If you are using cayenne powder, ½ teaspoon mixed into 8 ounces of water is a suggested dose. For capsules that contain the powder, a 450 mg capsule daily is typical. Side effects may include a risk of bleeding.

COENZYME Q10

Coenzyme Q10, or CoQ10 for short, is an antioxidant that is absolutely essential to life and one that is especially important for cardiovascular health. It is also known as ubiquinone (from ubiquitous), which indicates the fact that it can be found everywhere throughout the body. In the diet, CoQ10 is found primarily in meat and fish, but some is also in spinach, broccoli, whole grains, and peanuts. Nearly every cell in the body is capable of producing CoQ10, and so you might think that a deficiency would not be a problem. But you would be wrong.

CoQ10 has a lot of enemies: Extreme physical activity, use of statin drugs (which are used by tens of millions of people every day), aging (try to avoid that!), an overactive thyroid, low levels of the amino acid tyrosine, and deficiencies of several B vitamins all deplete CoQ10 levels. Low levels are often seen in patients who have chronic disease, such as heart conditions, Parkinson's disease, cancer, diabetes, and muscular dystrophies.

As a coenzyme, CoQ10 assists the mitochondria, which are the energy manufacturing centers of cells. Thus one of this coenzyme's main jobs is to help transform food into energy. Research shows, however, that it also plays a significant role in helping the heart. Given that the highest concentration of CoQ10 is in the heart, this fact comes as no surprise.

Why CoQ10 Is Heart-Healthy

Studies show that CoQ10 is a big supporter of cardiovascular health, as it is helpful in arrhythmia, congestive heart failure, coronary artery disease, high blood pressure, and in people who have heart surgery. As an antioxidant it converts heart-damaging free radicals into harmless substances and helps stop "bad" LDL cholesterol from forming plaque. Here's what the research shows.

- An article published in the April 2009 issue of *Medical Hypotheses* reported that CoQ10 has been used to effectively treat patients who have congestive heart failure because this antioxidant activates superoxide dismutase, which can lead to improved cardiac function, improvement in symptoms, and a better quality of life. The report also noted that the use of statins (which deplete CoQ10) along with CoQ10 appear to have a synergistic interaction on superoxide dismutase, which could benefit any patient who is taking statins.

- In a 2008 study, researchers studied the impact of administering CoQ10 to 46 patients who had hypertrophic cardiomyopathy compared with 41 matched controls who received conventional therapy. The CoQ10 patients received 200 mg daily and experienced a significant improvement in several indicators, including walking test, diastolic dysfunction, and posterior wall thickness. Ventricular tachycardia developed in four control patients but in none of the CoQ10 group.

- An Australian study reported that CoQ10 improved cardiac function in patients who had moderately severe dilated cardiomyopathy.

- The use of nanotechnology to help deliver CoQ10 is being investigated. Nanotechnology allows for substances to be reduced to nanoparticulate (extremely small) levels to allow the body to better utilize them. In an Indian study, researchers found that a nanoparticulate formulation of CoQ10 was effective in lowering high blood pressure in animal models and also required 60 percent less dosing than a traditional formulation.

- The heart-protective abilities of CoQ10 were explored in an Indiana study in which 100 mg of CoQ10 was given daily for 14 days before and 30 days after heart surgery. A control group received a placebo. Patients in both groups were deficient in CoQ10 before the study started. The CoQ10-treated patients showed improvement in cardiac function before surgery and significant improvement in length of recovery (3 to 5 days versus 15 to 30 in the control group). The CoQ10 preserved the myocardium during heart surgery and caused a significant improvement in cardiac pumping and left ventricular ejection fraction compared with controls.

How to Take CoQ10

A suggested dose of CoQ10 is 30 to 90 mg daily for healthy adults. Research studies of heart conditions typically use

90 to 200 mg daily, with some administering 100 mg three to four times daily.

Coenzyme Q10 should be taken with food that contains some oil to improve absorption. Because CoQ10 is fat soluble, it is not absorbed well from the gastrointestinal tract when taken on an empty stomach.

Coenzyme Q10 usually does not cause side effects. When they do occur, they may include mild, transient nausea, vomiting, diarrhea, loss of appetite, and heartburn. Rarely, serious adverse reactions such as fainting or dizziness (indicating low blood pressure), high liver enzyme levels, or allergic reactions (e.g., hives, difficulty breathing, itching, unexplained swelling) develop. If any of these symptoms occur, stop taking CoQ10 immediately and contact your physician.

D-RIBOSE

D-ribose is a carbohydrate that is produced naturally by the body and is used by all of the body's cells. It plays a critical role in the production of energy, and it is also necessary for the synthesis of nucleotides and for the formation of DNA and RNA molecules.

Supplements of D-ribose are often promoted for bodybuilders to help build endurance and improve performance, although there is no clear evidence that these supplements are effective for these purposes. However, D-ribose has been used successfully in treating cardiovascular disease as well as conditions such as chronic fatigue and symptoms associated with chronic fatigue syndrome.

The body typically makes enough D-ribose to handle the body's basic needs. The heart, skeletal muscle, brain, and nerve tissues can make only enough D-ribose to meet their own needs when they are not stressed. However, when blood and/or oxygen flow is deficient, especially chronically as in people who have heart disease, the body cannot make enough D-ribose to meet its needs, and the body becomes depleted.

Why D-Ribose Is Heart-Healthy

Several animal and human research studies have suggested that D-ribose benefits heart health and function by improving myocardial function after exercise and supporting cardiovascular metabolism. A brief summary of a few studies is below.

- In one study, a group of men who had stable coronary artery disease were given either 15 grams of D-ribose four times daily or a placebo. All the men underwent treadmill exercise tests on several different occasions to determine what effect, if any, D-ribose had on fatigue. The men who took the D-ribose took a significantly longer time to become fatigued than those who took a placebo.

- In another study, 15 healthy individuals were given 5 grams three times daily or D-ribose or placebo for three weeks. The investigators then conducted echocardiograms to determine heart function and found that those who took D-ribose had a "more efficient relaxation phase of the heart" and that the participants also reported a significant improvement in their quality of life than did subjects who took a placebo.

- In an animal study, researchers explored the ability of D-ribose to promote heart function. They administered D-ribose to rats and then studied their hearts for levels of ATP (adenosine triphosphate, a critical energy carrier in the body). Their findings indicate that D-ribose may enhance the preservation of ATP in the heart, which in turn promotes normal heart function.

How to Take D-Ribose

Studies show that an adequate dose of D-ribose usually provides results within a few days, and that even low doses can bring much relief. Although D-ribose is a safe supplement, it should be given by a knowledgeable health-care practitioner, as the doses can vary greatly depending on your heart condition.

For example, some experts recommend taking 5 grams (two teaspoons if using the powder) daily as a preventive measure and for athletes, while they suggest 10 to 115 grams for most people who have heart failure, peripheral vascular disease, stable angina, and individuals who are recovering from heart attack or heart surgery. If you have advanced heart failure, frequent angina, or dilated cardiomyopathy, your physician may recommend taking 15 to 30 grams daily.

Side effects are infrequent and mild. Because D-ribose can lower blood glucose levels, insulin-dependent diabetics should talk to their doctor before taking this supplement. Some people experience lightheadedness if they take 10 grams or more on an empty stomach. Taking D-ribose with meals or mixed into milk or juice can prevent this side effect.

GARLIC

Garlic is one of the most popular herbs enjoyed around the world for its culinary features. Fortunately, it is an effective healing herb as well, so you have the option of reaping its benefits from a supplement or on your dinner plate.

Garlic is a member of the *Allium* family, which also includes onions, leeks, and chives. It contains more than 200 chemicals, and one of the most beneficial is allicin, a sulfur compound. Allicin is formed in raw garlic whenever a clove is chopped, chewed, or crushed. This compound gives garlic its pungent taste and smell, and seems to have medicinal value as well.

Why Garlic Is Heart-Healthy

Garlic has been the subject of many clinical trials that have explored its role in heart disease. The list below contains just a few of these studies and their findings.

- In a 2007 review, investigators reported that garlic inhibits platelet aggregation through several means, one of which is by increasing the production of nitric oxide, and another by reducing the ability of platelets to bind to fibrinogen, which enhances the clumping of platelets. The researchers concluded that garlic inhibits platelet aggregation by several means and may have a role in preventing cardiovascular disease.

- In a meta-analysis performed at Hartford Hospital in Connecticut, investigators evaluated the results of 10 studies that included patients with and without elevated systolic blood pressure. They found that garlic reduced systolic blood pressure by 16.3 mmHg and diastolic blood pressure by 9.3 mmHg compared with placebo in patients who had elevated systolic blood pressure.

• A meta-analysis was conducted by experts at the University of Connecticut School of Pharmacy, who evaluated the results of 29 studies. They found that garlic significantly reduced total cholesterol but did not have an appreciable impact on low-density lipoprotein (LDL) or high-density lipoprotein (HDL) levels.

How to Take Garlic

The American Dietetic Association states that you need to take 600 to 900 mg (about 1 fresh garlic clove) per day to reap the potential health benefits. If you prefer to get all or most your garlic in a supplement, then you can consider the following doses. Keep in mind that if the smell of garlic on your breath bothers you (and others), some garlic supplements are odorless.

If you choose to take garlic oil, the suggested dose ranges from 4 to 12 mg daily. The European Scientific Cooperative on Phytotherapy recommends taking 3 to 5 mg allicin daily. That is equal to 1 clove or 0.5 to 1.0 gram of dried powder. The World Health Organization recommends taking 2 to 5 grams of fresh garlic, 0.4 to 12 grams of dried powder, 2 to 5 mg garlic oil, or 300 to 1,000 mg of garlic extract daily. The goal, according to the WHO, is to take an amount that gives you 2 to 5 mg of allicin daily.

GINGER

Ginger is a plant that originally comes from southeast Asia, but is now cultivated in Jamaica and other tropical areas. It is a very popular spice that is used around the world for both its culinary features and its medicinal value. In fact, the root (rhizome) of the ginger plant has been used in traditional Indian and Chinese medicine for more than 2,500 years to treat conditions such as diarrhea, colds, headache, and menstrual cramps. Your first thoughts of ginger may be of using it when baking or as a supplement to ease nausea. But ginger (*Zingiber officinalis*) also possesses some features that benefit the heart.

Why Ginger Is Heart-Healthy

Ginger is a rich source of antioxidants and also enhances the production of antioxidants in the body. In the scientific world, ginger is proving to have many heart-enhancing characteristics. We scoured the literature to find some of the most relevant ones for you.

- A review published in the January 2009 issue of the *International Journal of Cardiology* notes that recent trials suggest that ginger has considerable antiplatelet, blood-pressure-lowering, and cholesterol-lowering effects in laboratory and animal studies. Although there have been few human studies, dosages of 5 grams or more have shown significant antiplatelet effect. The authors note that more human studies are needed and if the results are positive, ginger could become not only a less expensive alternative to conventional medications but one that has significantly fewer side effects as well.

- In a 2002 animal study, researchers evaluated the ability of ginger to lower cholesterol and triglycerides. They found that high doses (500 mg/kg) significantly reduced cholesterol but did not reduce triglyceride levels. Ginger also had a beneficial effect on inflammation and platelet accumulation, both very important for heart health.

- Ginger dissolves fibrin and reduces the body's ability to make this substance. Fibrin is a fibrous protein that attracts and entangles cells and platelets, which leads to the formation of a clot. If you have a history of stroke or atherosclerosis, ginger may help prevent a recurrence of these conditions.

- In a 2006 study, researchers found that a combination of 1 gram of ginger along with 10 mg nifedipine (a drug used to treat high blood pressure) can be an important combination for people who have cardiovascular and cerebrovascular complications associated with platelet aggregation.

How to Take Ginger

Ginger supplements are available as tablets, capsules, liquid extract, tincture, fresh and dried root, and tea. Look for supplements that contain ginger's active ingredients, which include gingerols (which give ginger its odor and flavor) and shogaols.

The recommended doses range from 1 to 4 grams daily, divided into smaller doses. Side effects from ginger supplements are usually mild and may include nausea, stomach upset, belching, bloating, or heartburn. You can reduce the possibility of experiencing these side effects by taking ginger capsules rather than powder. Do not take ginger if you have a bleeding disorder or are taking anti-platelet medication, or if you have gallstones.

GINKGO BILOBA

Ginkgo biloba is one of the oldest herbal remedies known to humankind, dating back five thousand years or more. Traditionally, ginkgo remedies were made mainly from the fruit and nuts of the ginkgo tree to treat conditions ranging from bedwetting to respiratory problems, low sexual energy, cancer, gonorrhea, asthma, and urinary tract infections. The leaves were used much less often, and then only for a few conditions.

Today, however, ginkgo biloba leaf extracts are one of the most popular herbal remedies, especially in Germany and other European countries. Ginkgo stepped into the spotlight in the United States in the late 1990s when scientists discovered that it may benefit people who have Alzheimer's disease. Since that time, researchers have continued to uncover other advantages of ginkgo biloba supplements, including heart function.

Why Ginkgo Biloba Is Heart-Healthy

The main contribution ginkgo biloba makes to furthering heart health is by improving blood circulation. It may also act as an antioxidant and help reduce free-radical damage to the heart.

- Atherosclerosis involves the buildup of plaque inside the arteries and other blood vessels, which reduces blood flow and the ability of the body to heal itself from free-radical damage. Ginkgo biloba improves blood flow and may help promote healing of the blood vessels.

- Several studies, including one performed at Stanford University Medical School in California, suggest that ginkgo biloba causes some improvement in leg pain associated with intermittent claudication and peripheral artery disease. In the Stanford study, for example, participants took 300 mg per day of ginkgo biloba or placebo for four months. Patients who took the ginkgo experienced a modest increase in walking time and pain-free walking time compared with patients in the placebo group.

- Ginkgo biloba can help improve blood flow. In a 2008 study, patients with coronary artery disease were randomly assigned to receive either ginkgo biloba extract or placebo for two weeks. Using Doppler echocardiography, the researchers found that patients who had taken ginkgo biloba experienced a significant improvement in blood flow on the distal left anterior descending coronary artery.

How to Take Ginkgo Biloba

Ginkgo biloba supplements are available as capsules, tablets, and liquid extract. A typical dosage is 80 to 150 mg daily. Look for products standardized to 24 percent to 25 percent ginkgo flavone glycosides and 6 percent terpine lactones.

Ginkgo biloba is generally well tolerated when taken as recommended for up to six months. Mild symptoms may include headache, nausea, and intestinal discomfort.

HAWTHORN

The hawthorn plant is a thorny shrub that grows on hillsides and wooded areas throughout North America, North Africa, Europe, and Western Asia. After the shrub flowers each May, the bright red berries, called haws, appear. The leaves are usually shiny and can grow in different sizes and shapes.

Hawthorn fruit was first recognized as a treatment for heart disease in the first century. It has also been used to relieve digestive and kidney problems. Both the leaves and flowers are used to make liquid extracts, usually with water and alcohol. Dry extracts are placed into capsules and tablets.

Why Hawthorn Is Heart-Healthy

Hawthorn has been well-known as an herb that helps the heart. The credit for this benefit has been given to the bioflavonoid complexes found in the leaves, berries, and flowers. These include oligomeric procyanidins (OPCs), quercetin, vitexin, and hyperoside. These phytonutrients have been studied widely. Here's what the study results show.

- Recent animal studies show that hawthorn herb may lower cholesterol levels by enhancing the body's ability to metabolize the lipid. Scientists then used hawthorn in human studies and came up with similar results.

- In a 2008 study published in the *Cochrane Database of Systematic Reviews,* experts looked at the use of hawthorn in 14 randomized, double-blind, placebo-controlled trials. They found that use of hawthorn significantly increased exercise tolerance and also resulted in a significant improvement in shortness of breath and fatigue.

- Some experts believe hawthorn contains elements that act directly on the heart muscle to increase the force of the organ's beat and also relaxes the arteries around the heart.

- A study published in the *European Journal of Heart Failure* reported on the results of a randomized, double-blind, placebo-controlled, multicenter trial in which 2,681 people with congestive heart failure were given 900 mg hawthorn (or a placebo) per day for 24 months. The authors concluded that hawthorn has the potential to reduce the incidence of sudden cardiac death, at least in patients with less compromised left ventricular function.

How to Take Hawthorn

Look for hawthorn supplements that are standardized to contain 2.2 percent bioflavonoids or 18.75 percent oligomeric procyanidins. The suggested dosage of dried extract is 160 to 900 mg daily, divided into two to three doses if you have congestive heart failure. Do not expect instant results: When taking hawthorn for angina or heart failure, you will need to take it for at least two weeks before you notice some effect. For maximum benefit, you must take hawthorn for at least four to eight weeks.

If you take too much hawthorn, you may experience dizziness, hypotension, cardiac arrhythmias, tremors, and sedation. Use of hawthorn may enhance the activity of digoxin, a medication that is often used by people who have irregular heart rhythms. Do not take hawthorn if you are pregnant or nursing.

OMEGA-3 FATTY ACIDS

Omega-3 fatty acids are called essential because while they are essential to human health, the body cannot manufacture them. Therefore it is necessary to get them from food and/or supplements. Most of the foods that are good sources of omega-3 fatty acids are fish, such as salmon, tuna, and halibut, along with some nut oils.

The American Heart Association recommends eating fish at least twice per week. However, because many people do not like fish or eat very little of it, omega-3 fatty acid supplements may be needed, especially for the prevention and treatment of heart disease.

Omega-3 fats are also important for the production of hormone-like substances called prostaglandins. Prostaglandins help regulate critical functions, such as blood pressure, blood clotting, and inflammatory responses, all of which are important in heart disease and heart function.

There are three main types of omega-3 fatty acids in foods: alpha-linolenic acid (ALA), eicosapentaenoic acid

(EPA), and docosahexaenoic acid (DHA). If you eat foods that contain ALA, the body converts it to EPA and DHA, because the body can more readily use them in this form.

Why Omega-3 Fatty Acids Are Heart-Healthy

Research shows that omega-3 fatty acids help prevent risk factors associated with heart disease, cancer, and other serious conditions. In fact, symptoms of omega-3 fatty acid deficiency include heart problems and poor circulation, as well as poor memory, fatigue, mood swings, and dry skin. Here's what some of the studies show.

- A 2007 study found that EPA may help prevent nonfatal heart problems in people who have high cholesterol. The study included more than 18,600 adults who had high cholesterol (including 3,660 who had a history of coronary artery disease). The participants were followed for more than four years, during which time they took either statin drugs or statins plus EPA supplements. The investigators found that 2.8 percent of the patients who took EPA plus statins experienced a major coronary event, compared with 3.5 percent of those who took only statins, a 19 percent difference. The scientists also noted that the advantage of taking EPA applied only to the patients with a known history of coronary artery disease. The researchers concluded that EPA is promising for preventing heart problems in patients who have high cholesterol.

- A study published in the *American Journal of Clinical Nutrition* evaluated the role of omega-3 fatty acids in ischemic heart disease and sudden cardiac death. The study examined the effects of EPA and DHA in 38 adults who had high cholesterol. The patients were randomly assigned to take either an EPA supplement, a DHA supplement, or a placebo for seven weeks. At the end of the study, patients in the EPA group had a 36 percent improvement and those in the DHA group had a 27 percent improvement in arterial compliance (a measure of how elastic an artery is, as stiff arteries can lead to hypertension). Patients in the placebo group showed no change. These results indicate that omega-3 fatty acids may help prevent ischemic heart disease and sudden cardiac death.

• A 2009 review study from the University of Guelph noted that omega-3 fatty acids in the form of EPA and DHA lower triglyceride levels, improve HDL cholesterol levels, reduce the risk for progression of coronary atherosclerosis, and lower the risk of sudden cardiac death. The reviewers also point out that DHA supplementation reduces blood pressure and resting heart rates. They also note that specific recommendations for the optimal doses for DHA and EPA have not yet been determined.

How to Take Omega-3 Fatty Acids

Omega-3 fatty acid supplements are available as bottled liquids and as softgels. The most popular omega-3 supplements are flaxseed oil (a rich source of ALA) and cod liver oil (rich source of EPA and DHA).

Although a definitive dosage for EPA and DHA has not been determined, the World Health Organization and other health agencies recommend taking 0.3 to 0.5 grams daily of EPA plus DHA and 0.8 to 1.1 grams of ALA. When purchasing omega-3 fatty acid supplements, choose certified organic products that have been refrigerated and are packaged in a dark glass container, as these oils are highly sensitive to damage from heat, light, and oxygen. If possible, choose a supplement that contains vitamin E, which helps prevent the fatty acids from becoming rancid.

RED YEAST RICE

Red yeast rice is the product of yeast *(Monascus purpureus)* that is grown on rice. It contains substances known collectively as monacolins, which have been shown to inhibit the synthesis of cholesterol. One specific monacolin, called monacolin K, is also known as lovastatin (brand name, Mevacor), a common statin drug used to lower cholesterol levels.

A natural over-the-counter supplement called Cholestin™ contains red yeast rice, and although it is effective, there has been a legal dispute over whether the product should be classified as a drug or a dietary supplement. That's because unlike prescription drugs, herbal remedies are not subject to formal safety evaluation by the FDA. Some medical professionals are concerned that some red yeast extracts may contain an unsafe dose of lovastatin or perhaps even unknown contaminants.

Why Red Yeast Rice Is Heart-Healthy

When it comes to matters of the heart, red yeast rice seems to shine in the cholesterol department, but it has some other advantages as well. Here's what the studies show.

- In a randomized, controlled study, ~~62 patients~~ who had high cholesterol and who could not take statins because of side effects were given red yeast rice (1,800 mg) or a placebo twice daily for 24 weeks. Patients who took the red yeast rice experienced a significantly lower LDL cholesterol level after 12 and 24 weeks of treatment than did the placebo group. Levels of HDL and triglycerides did not differ significantly between the two groups; nor did weight loss.

- In a large review, investigators evaluated a study in which 4,870 patients participated. The results of the trial showed a 46 percent reduction in nonfatal myocardial infarction and coronary death among participants who took red yeast rice supplement.

How to Take Red Yeast Rice

The suggested dose of red yeast rice is three 600-mg capsules daily. This is the dosage used in the latest study (*Annals of Internal Medicine*, 2009). You should note, however, that because herbal supplements are not regulated by the Food and Drug Administration (FDA), consumers cannot be certain they are getting the amount of product listed on the supplement label.

For example, in the 2009 study, some of the investigators analyzed 12 different brands of red yeast rice and found a hundredfold difference in the concentrations of the product. Therefore, it is important to purchase red yeast rice supplements from a reputable manufacturer and to also consult with your physician about the product you choose.

If you have liver disease or are at risk for liver disease, or if you have an acute infection or kidney disease, you should avoid taking red yeast rice supplements. Women who are pregnant or breastfeeding also should not take this supplement. If you experience muscle tenderness or pain while using red yeast rice, stop taking the supplement and consult with your doctor.

RESVERATROL

Since the turn of the new millennium, there has been a growing interest in a polyphenol called resveratrol, which is found in red wine, grapes, peanuts, and some berries. One reason for the interest is that resveratrol appears to offer many benefits when it comes to heart health.

Resveratrol is produced by some plants in response to stress, fungal infections, ultraviolet radiation, or injury. Scientists first became curious about resveratrol in 1992 when it was discovered in red wine, and some experts speculated that this phytonutrient might help explain the "French Paradox": why the French can smoke and eat foods high in saturated fat yet experience a low rate of death from coronary heart disease.

Why Resveratrol Is Heart-Healthy

Numerous studies have been conducted and more are in process to identify the ways resveratrol can benefit the heart. Thus far, scientists have made the following discoveries.

- Resveratrol may protect the heart by reducing the impact of cardiac fibrosis, which is hardening of the heart muscle. In an animal study, researchers found that treating heart cells with resveratrol prevented the damaging activity of a hormone called angiotensin II. Angiotensin II causes the heart muscle to stiffen, which forces the heart to work harder, resulting in damage to the myocardium.

- In a study performed at New York Medical College, the investigators found that resveratrol blocks the accumulation of platelets, which is important in preventing heart attack and stroke.

- Resveratrol stimulates the production of endothelial nitric oxide, which is related to heart disease prevention. This is how it works: Nitric oxide is a substance that helps prevent clogging of arteries. When nitric oxide levels increase in the endothelium (the innermost layer of cells inside the arteries), they protect the artery walls and maintain relaxed arteries. When nitric oxide is unable to perform this function, the risk of cardiovascular disease increases.

- Resveratrol inhibits the proliferation of vascular smooth muscle cells. This is an important role in the progression of atherosclerosis.

How to Take Resveratrol
Resveratrol supplements are available in capsules and tablets. Most resveratrol supplements contain extracts of

the root of *Polygonum cuspidatum,* which is also known as Hu Zhang. Red grape and red wine extracts that contain resveratrol and other polyphenols are also available. Resveratrol supplements typically contain 10 to 50 mg, but the effective doses for prevention and treatment of heart disease and related conditions is not known.

Thus far researchers have not identified any significant side effects or toxicity associated with the use of resveratrol. Because much still is not known about the effects of resveratrol, women who are pregnant or nursing should not take the supplement.

TURMERIC (CURCUMIN)

Turmeric is a native plant of southern India and Indonesia, where the people have harvested it for more than 5,000 years. It has long been a popular member of both Ayurvedic and Chinese medicine, whose practitioners have used it for its anti-inflammatory properties. Arab traders carried turmeric to Europe in the thirteenth century, and it gradually made its way to other countries over the centuries. Today the main producers of turmeric include India, Indonesia, China, the Philippines, Taiwan, Haiti, and Jamaica.

Turmeric comes from the root of the *Curcuma longa* plant and contains a pigment called curcumin, which is believed to be the main active ingredient in turmeric. Although curcumin has anti-inflammatory effects that rival those of several prescription and over-the-counter drugs, it has minimal side effects. Turmeric has a bitter, peppery flavor and is one of the primary ingredients in curry.

Why Turmeric Is Heart-Healthy

In addition to turmeric's anti-inflammatory benefits, it also has demonstrated heart-friendly advantages. We give a few examples here.

- Studies indicate that curcumin may prevent oxidation of cholesterol. Because oxidized cholesterol damages blood vessels and promotes development of plaque that leads to stroke and heart attack, the use of curcumin may prevent atherosclerosis and heart disease. In one study, 10 healthy participants consumed 500 mg of curcumin daily for seven days. At the end of the seven days, total cholesterol levels declined 11.63 percent, blood levels of oxidized cholesterol fell 33 percent, and the level of good cholesterol (HDL) rose 29 percent.

- Turmeric can lower cholesterol because of how curcumin communicates with the liver. Curcumin signals liver cells to increase the production of mRNA (messenger proteins) that direct the creation of receptors for LDL cholesterol. The more LDL receptors the body has, the more LDL cholesterol can be eliminated from the body. A study found that the number of LDL-receptor mRNA increased sevenfold in liver cells treated with curcumin.

- Preliminary research indicates that curcumin may help the heart by lowering blood pressure and preventing blood clots. Further study is needed to verify these findings.

How to Take Turmeric/Curcumin

Both curcumin and turmeric are available in capsule and liquid extract form, and turmeric is available as dried root. Doses range from 450 mg of curcumin capsules to 3 grams of turmeric root daily, divided into several doses. When shopping for curcumin supplements, look for products that contain at least 95 percent turmeric extracts.

Turmeric may cause stomach upset, especially if taken in high doses or taken for a long period of time. Other side effects may include heartburn, diarrhea, or nausea. If you have a bleeding disorder or take drugs that may increase the risk of bleeding, consult your doctor before taking turmeric or curcumin.

CHAPTER 6

Seven Days of Delicious Heart-Healthy Eating

So far, we have explained why it's critical to follow a healthy diet if you want to help prevent heart disease or manage it if you have a heart condition. But just how easy *is* it to eat a heart-healthy diet?

Rather than tell you how easy it can be, we will let you make that discovery for yourself in this chapter. Here we provide you with seven days of menu ideas and recipes. Nearly all of the items in the menus incorporate the heart-healthy foods you read about in chapter 4, as well as the recipes from that chapter.

For example, Monday morning breakfast includes "Almond Banana Beverage," the lunch suggestion is for "Gazpacho," and the dinner options include "Greens and Pasta" and "Red Wine Soup." Each recipe is in italics for easy identification.

Many of the recipes contain more than one heart-healthy food item. A few of the menu items do not have recipes, but they do include the heart-healthy foods that we discussed in chapter 4, and they are very easy to prepare. For example, for one lunch we suggest a whole-grain pita stuffed with tuna, tomato, and "Flax Salsa": a heart-healthy sandwich that doesn't require a recipe to prepare—the Flax Salsa is an option, but a delicious one! In a few cases we suggest a menu item on more than one occasion. Many of the recipes are great as leftovers, and that means you don't have to cook for that meal!

So get ready to enjoy some delicious and easy-to-prepare treats that your heart will thank you for.

MONDAY
Breakfast
Almond Banana Beverage
Whole-grain bagel with whole fruit spread
Herbal tea

Lunch
Gazpacho
Whole grain crackers
Fresh strawberries

Dinner
Greens and Pasta
Red Wine Soup
Sparking water

TUESDAY
Breakfast
Poached Papaya
Whole-grain bagel with Figgy Salsa
Herbal tea

Lunch
Eggplant Stew
Kiwi Blend

Dinner
Spicy Tuna
Grilled Sweet Potatoes
Tomato, cucumber, and onion salad with Olive Oil/Lemon
Dressing
Sparkling flavored water

WEDNESDAY
Breakfast
Scrambled egg whites with your favorite vegetables
Plum Compote
Green tea

Lunch
White turkey slices on whole-grain bread
Four Pepper Salad
Sparkling water

Dinner
Tofu Burgers (whole-grain optional)
Baked Onions and Potatoes
Simply Asparagus
Tomato juice

THURSDAY
Breakfast
Almond Blueberry Oatmeal

Fresh berries
Green tea

Lunch
Zucchini and Walnuts
Frozen Mango Magic
Herbal tea

Dinner
Baked Chicken breast
Bean and Kale Salad
Middle Eastern Squash
Green tea

FRIDAY
Breakfast
Berry Berry Sundae
Pomegranate Punch

Lunch
Tabouli with whole-grain crackers
Fresh plums
Tomato juice

Dinner
Lemon Broiled Tempeh
Rainbow Barley Salad
Carrots with Kick
Herbal tea

SATURDAY
Breakfast
Whole-grain waffles with Figgy Salsa
Banana Blueberry Smoothie

Lunch
Rainbow Barley Salad
Chocolate-Dipped Strawberries
Sparkling water

Dinner
Relished Salmon
Broccoli and Sweet Potatoes
Orange and Red Salad
Herbal tea

SUNDAY
Breakfast
Baked Apple with Crunch
Whole-grain toast with no-fat cream cheese
Green tea

Lunch
Brown Rice and Asparagus
Green Tea Smoothie

Dinner
Lentil Soup
Greens, tomatoes, cucumbers, and onion salad with Olive Oil/Lemon Dressing
Whole-grain roll
Sparkling flavored water

SNACKS

Green Tea Smoothie
Just the Flax Salsa with vegetable slices
No-fat yogurt with fresh fruit
Apricot Hats
Chocolate-Dipped Strawberries
Figgy Salsa with fresh apple slices
What's Shaking Shake

APPENDIX

Notes

Introduction
Mente A et al. A systematic review of the evidence supporting a causal link between dietary factors and coronary heart disease. *Arch Intern Med* 2009 Apr 13; 169(7): 659–69.

Chapter 3
Boraita PA. Exercise as the cornerstone of cardiovascular prevention. *Rev Esp Cardiol* 2008 May; 61(5): 514–28.

Williams PT, Hoffman KM. Optimal body weight for the prevention of coronary heart disease in normal-weight physically active men. *Obesity* (Silver Spring) 2009 Jul; 17(7): 1428–34.

Chapter 4
ALMONDS
Jenkins DJ et al. Dose response of almonds on coronary heart disease risk factors: blood lipids, oxidized low-density

lipoproteins, lipoprotein(a), homocysteine, and pulmonary nitric oxide: a randomized, controlled, crossover trial. *Circulation* 2002 Sep 10; 106(11): 1327–32.

Milbury PE et al. Determination of flavonoids and phenolics and their distribution in almonds. *Agric Food Chem* 2006 Jul 12; 54(14): 5027–33.

APPLES
Mink PJ et al. Flavonoid intake and cardiovascular disease mortality: a prospective study in postmenopausal women. *Am J Clin Nutr* 2007 Mar; 85(3): 895–909.

APRICOTS
Kohlmeyer L, Kark JD, Gomez-Garcia E, et al. Lycopene and myocardial infarction risk in the EUROMIC study. *Am J Epidemiol* 1997; 146: 618–26.

Osganian SK et al. Dietary carotenoids and risk of coronary artery disease in women. *Am J Clin Nutr* 2003 Jun; 77(6): 1390–99.

ASPARAGUS
Karthick M et al. Preventive effect of rutin, a bioflavonoid, on lipid peroxides and antioxidants in isoproterenol-induced myocardial infarction in rats. *J Pharm Pharmacol* 2006 May; 58(5): 701–7.

da Silva RR et al. Hypocholesterolemic effect of naringin and rutin flavonoids. *Arch Latinoam Nutr* 2001 Sep; 51(3): 258–64.

Wang M et al. Quantification of protodioscin and rutin in

asparagus shoots by LC/MS and HPLC methods. *J Agric Food Chem* 2003 Oct 8; 51(21): 6132–36.

BANANAS
Ascherio A et al. Intake of potassium, magnesium, calcium, and fiber and risk of stroke among US men. *Circulation* 1998 Sep 22; 98(12): 1198–204.

Bazzano LA et al. Dietary fiber intake and reduced risk of coronary heart disease in US men and women: the National Health and Nutrition Examination Survey I Epidemiologic Follow-up Study. *Arch Intern Med* 2003 Sep 8; 163(16): 1897–904.

BARLEY
Ames NP, Rhymer CR. Issues surrounding health claims for barley. *J Nutr* 2008 Jun; 138(6): 1237S–43S.

Food and Drug Administration, HHS. Food labeling: health claims; soluble dietary fiber from certain foods and coronary heart disease. Final rule. *Fed Regist* 2006 May 22; 71(98): 29248–50.

Schnabel R et al. Selenium supplementation improves antioxidant capacity in vitro and in vivo in patients with coronary artery disease. The Selenium Therapy in Coronary Artery Disease Patients (SETCAP) Study. *Am Heart J* 2008 Dec; 156(6): 1201.e1–11.

BELL PEPPERS
Bazzano LA et al. Dietary intake of folate and risk of stroke in US men and women: NHANES I Epidemiologic Follow-up Study. *Stroke* 2002 May; 33(5): 1183–89.

Sesso HD et al. Plasma lycopene, other carotenoids, and retinol and the risk of cardiovascular disease in women. *Am J Clin Nutr* 2004 Jan; 79(1): 47–53.

BERRIES
Erlund I et al. Favorable effects of berry consumption on platelet function, blood pressure, and HDL cholesterol. *Am J Clin Nutr* 2008 Feb; 87(2): 323–31.

Youdim KA et al. Potential role of dietary flavonoids in reducing microvascular endothelium vulnerability to oxidative and inflammatory insults. *J Nutr Biochem* 2002 May; 13(5): 282–88.

Youdim KA et al. Polyphenolics enhance red blood cell resistance to oxidative stress: in vitro and in vivo. *Biochim Biophys Acta* 2000 Sep 1; 1523(1): 117–22.

BROCCOLI
Lin J et al. Dietary intakes of flavonols and flavones and coronary heart disease in US women. *Am J Epidemiol* 2007 Jun 1; 165(11): 1305–13.

Maiyoh GK et al. Cruciferous indole-3-carbinol inhibits apolipoprotein B secretion in HepG2 cells 1–3. *J Nutr* 2007; 37:2185–89.

Mukherjee S et al. Broccoli: a unique vegetable that protects mammalian hearts through the redox cycling of the thioredoxin superfamily. *J Agric Food Chem* 2008 Jan 23; 56(2): 609–17.

BROWN RICE

Anderson JW et al. Whole grain foods and heart disease risk. *J Am Coll Nutr* 2000 Jun; 19(3 Suppl): 291S–99S.

Most MM et al. Rice bran oil, not fiber, lowers cholesterol in humans. *Am J Clin Nutr* 2005 Jan; 81(1): 64–68. 2005.

van Dam RM, et al. Dietary calcium and magnesium, major food sources, and risk of type 2 diabetes in U.S. Black women. *Diabetes Care* 2006 Oct; 29(10): 2238–43.

Vanharanta M et al. Risk of cardiovascular disease-related and all-cause death according to serum concentrations of enterolactone: Kuopio Ischaemic Heart Disease Risk Factor Study. *Arch Intern Med* 2003 May 12; 163(9): 1099–104.

BULGAR

Pereira MA et al. Dietary fiber and risk of coronary heart disease. *Arch Intern Med* 2004; 164: 370–76.

CARROTS

Mente A et al. A systematic review of the evidence supporting a causal link between dietary factors and coronary heart disease. *Arch Intern Med* 2009 Apr 13; 169(7): 659–69.

Nicolle C et al. Effect of carrot intake on cholesterol metabolism and on antioxidant status in cholesterol-fed rat. *Eur J Nutr* 2003 Oct; 42(5): 254–61.

Ye A, Song H. Antioxidant vitamins intake and the risk of coronary heart disease: meta-analysis of cohort studies. *Eur J Cardiovasc Prev Rehabil* 2008 Feb; 15(1): 26–34.

DARK CHOCOLATE

Engler MB et al. Flavonoid-rich dark chocolate improves endothelial function and increases plasma epicatechin concentrations in healthy adults. *J Am Coll Nutr* 2004 Jun; 23(3): 197–204.

Rizzo M, Berneis K. Recent insights on dark chocolate consumption and cardiovascular risk. *South Med J* 2008 Dec; 101(12): 1194.

Serafini M et al. Plasma antioxidants from chocolate. *Nature* 2003 Aug 28; 424: 1013.

Taubert D et al. Chocolate and blood pressure in elderly individuals with isolated systolic hypertension. *JAMA* 2003 Aug 27; 290(8): 1029–30.

EGGPLANT

Jorge PA et al. Effect of eggplant on plasma lipid levels, lipidic peroxidation and reversion of endothelial dysfunction in experimental hypercholesterolemia. *Arq Bras Cardiol* 1998 Feb; 70(2): 87–91.

Kimura Y et al. Protective effects of dietary nasunin on paraquat-induced oxidative stress in rats. *Biosci Biotechnol Biochem* 1999 May; 63(5): 799–804.

Noda Y et al. Antioxidant activity of nasunin, an anthocyanin in eggplant peels. *Toxicology* 2000 Aug 7; 148(2–3): 119–23.

FIGS

Appel LJ et al. A clinical trial of the effects of dietary patterns on blood pressure. DASH Collaborative Research Group. *N Engl J Med* 1997 Apr 17; 336(16): 1117–24.

Canal JR et al. A chloroform extract obtained from a decoction of Ficus carica leaves improves the cholesterol-aemic status of rats with streptozotocin-induced diabetes. *Acta Physiol Hung* 2000; 87(1): 71–6.

Ludwig DS et al. Dietary fiber, weight gain, and cardiovascular disease risk factors in young adults. *JAMA* 1999 Oct 27; 282(16): 1539–46.

FLAXSEED

Bazzano LA et al. Dietary fiber intake and reduced risk of coronary heart disease in US men and women: the National Health and Nutrition Examination Survey I Epidemiologic Follow-up Study. *Arch Intern Med* 2003 Sep 8; 163(16): 1897–904.

Ueshima H et al. Food omega-3 fatty acid intake of individuals (total, linolenic acid, long-chain) and their blood pressure. INTERMAP Study. *Hypertension* 2007 Jun 4.

GREENS

Nicolle C et al. Health effect of vegetable-based diet: lettuce consumption improves cholesterol metabolism and antioxidant status in the rat. *Clin Nutr* 2004 Aug; 23(4): 605–14.

Voutilainen S et al. Carotenoids and cardiovascular health. *Am J Clin Nutr* 2006 Jun; 83(6): 1265–71.

Ye Z, Song H. Antioxidant vitamins intake and the risk of coronary heart disease: meta-analysis of cohort studies. *Eur J Cardiovasc Prev Rehabil* 2008 Feb; 15(1): 26–34.

GREEN TEA
Alexopoulos N et al. The acute effect of green tea consumption on endothelial function in healthy individuals. *Eur J Cardiovasc Prev Rehabil* 2008; 16: 300–05.

Nantz MP et al. Standardized capsule of Camellia sinensis lowers cardiovascular risk factors in a randomized, double-blind, placebo-controlled study. *Nutrition* 2009 Feb; 25(2): 147–54.

KIWI
Duttaroy A, Jørgensen A. Effects of kiwi fruit consumption on platelet aggregation and plasma lipids in healthy human volunteers. *Platelets* 2004 Aug; 15(5): 287–292.

Kurl S et al. Plasma vitamin C modifies the association between hypertension and risk of stroke. *Stroke* 2002 Jun; 33(6): 1568–73.

LENTILS
Bazzano LA et al. Dietary intake of folate and risk of stroke in US men and women: NHANES I Epidemiologic Follow-up Study. *Stroke* 2002 May; 33(5): 1183–89.

Davies M, Ghosh A. Towards evidence based emergency medicine: best BETs from the Manchester Royal Infirmary. Prophylactic magnesium in myocardial infarction. *Emerg Med J* 2001 Mar; 18(2):119–20.

Kharb S, Singh V. Magnesium deficiency potentiates free radical production associated with myocardial infarction. *J Assoc Physicians India* 2000 May; 48(5): 484–85.

McIntosh M, Miller C. A diet containing food rich in soluble and insoluble fiber improves glycemic control and reduces hyperlipidemia among patients with type 2 diabetes mellitus. *Nutr Rev* 2001 Feb; 59(2): 52–55.

Menotti A et al. Food intake patterns and 25-year mortality from coronary heart disease: cross-cultural correlations in the Seven Countries Study. The Seven Countries Study Research Group. *Eur J Epidemiol* 1999 Jul; 15(6): 507–15.

Sueda S et al. Magnesium deficiency in patients with recent myocardial infarction and provoked coronary artery spasm. *Jpn Circ J* 2001 Jul; 65(7): 643–48.

Touyz RM. Role of magnesium in the pathogenesis of hypertension. *Mol Aspects Med* 2003 Feb 6; 24(1–3): 107–36.

MANGO

Egert S et al. Quercetin reduces systolic blood pressure and plasma oxidized low-density lipoprotein concentrations in overweight subjects with a high-cardiovascular disease risk phenotype: a double-blinded, placebo-controlled cross-over study. *Br J Nutr* 2009 Apr 30: 1–10.

Ghosh D, Scheepens A. Vascular action of polyphenols. *Mol Nutr Food Res* 2009 Mar; 53(3): 322–31.

Rocha Ribeiro SM et al. Antioxidant in mango (Mangifera indica L) pulp. *Plant Foods Hum Nutr* 2007 Mar; 62(1): 13–17.

Vita JA. Polyphenols and cardiovascular disease: effects on endothelial and platelet function. *Am J Clin Nutr* 2005 Jan; 81(1): 292S–97S.

OATMEAL

Chen CY et al. Avenanthramides phenolic acids from oats are bioavailable and act synergistically with vitamin C to enhance hamster and human LDL resistance to oxidation. *J Nutr* 2004 Jun; 134(6): 1459–66. 2004.

Djousse L, Gaziano JM. Breakfast cereals and risk of heart failure in the Physicians Health Study I. *Arch Intern Med* 2007 Oct 22; 167(19): 2080–85.

Erkkila AT et al. Cereal fiber and whole-grain intake are associated with reduced progression of coronary-artery atherosclerosis in postmenopausal women with coronary artery disease. *Am Heart J* 2005 Jul; 150(1): 94–101.

Liu L et al. The antiatherogenic potential of oat phenolic compounds. *Atherosclerosis* 2004 Jul; 175(1): 39–49.

OLIVE OIL

Aguilera CM et al. Protective effect of monounsaturated and polyunsaturated fatty acids on the development of cardiovascular disease. *Nutr Hosp* 2001 May–Jun; 16(3): 78–91.

Covas MI. Bioactive effects of olive oil phenolic compounds in humans: reduction of heart disease factors and oxidative damage. *Inflammopharmacology* 2008 Oct; 16(5): 216–18.

Covas MI et al. EUROLIVE Study Group. The effect of polyphenols in olive oil on heart disease risk factors: a randomized trial. *Ann Intern Med* 2006 Sep 5; 145(5): 333–41.

Covas MI. Olive oil and the cardiovascular system. *Pharmacol Res* 2007 Mar; 55(3): 175–86.

Kontogianni MD et al. The impact of olive oil consumption pattern on the risk of acute coronary syndromes: The CARDIO2000 case-control study. *Clin Cardiol* 2007 Mar; 30(3): 125–29.

Ruano J et al. Intake of phenol-rich virgin olive oil improves the postprandial prothrombotic profile in hypercholesterolemic patients. *Am J Clin Nutr* 2007 Aug; 86(2): 341–46.

Ruano J et al. Phenolic content of virgin olive oil improves ischemic reactive hyperemia in hypercholesterolemic patients. *J Am Coll Cardiol* 2005 Nov 15; 46(10): 1864–68.

Teres S et al. Oleic acid content is responsible for the reduction in blood pressure induced by olive oil. *Proc Natl Acad Sci USA* 2008 Sep 16; 105(37): 13811–16.

ONIONS

Huxley RR, Neil HAW. The relation between dietary flavonol intake and coronary heart disease mortality: a meta-analysis of prospective cohort studies. *Eur J Clin Nutr* 2003; 57: 904–8.

Yang J, et al. Varietal differences in phenolic content and antioxidant and antiproliferative activities of onions. *J Agric Food Chem* 2004 Nov 3; 52(22): 6787–93.

ORANGES
Galati EM et al. Biological effects of hesperidin, a citrus flavonoid. (Note I): antiinflammatory and analgesic activity. *Farmaco* 1994 Nov; 40(11): 709–12.

Galati EM et al. Biological effects of hesperidin, a citrus flavonoid. (Note III): antihypertensive and diuretic activity in rat. *Farmaco* 1996 Mar; 51(3): 219–21.

Kurl S et al. Plasma vitamin C modifies the association between hypertension and risk of stroke. *Stroke* 2002 Jun; 33(6): 1568–73.

Kurowska EM, Manthey JA. Hypolipidemic effects and absorption of citrus polymethoxylated flavones in hamsters with diet-induced hypercholesterolemia. *J Agric Food Chem* 2004 May 19; 52(10): 2879–86.

PAPAYA
Jarvik GP et al. Vitamin C and E intake is associated with increased paraoxonase activity. *Arterioscler Thromb Vasc Biol* 2002 Aug 1; 22(8): 1329–33.

PLUMS
Gallaher CM, Gallaher DD. Dried plums (prunes) reduce atherosclerosis lesion area in apolipoprotein E-deficient mice. *Br J Nutr* 2009 Jan; 101(2): 233–39.

Kurl S, Tuomainen TP, Laukkanen JA et al. Plasma vitamin C modifies the association between hypertension and risk of stroke. *Stroke* 2002 Jun; 33(6): 1568–73.

POMEGRANATES

Aviram M et al. Pomegranate juice consumption for 3 years by patients with carotid artery stenosis reduces common carotid intima-media thickness, blood pressure and LDL oxidation. *Clin Nutr* 2004 Jun; 23(3): 423–33.

Basu A, Penugonda K. Pomegranate juice: a heart-healthy fruit juice. *Nutr Rev* 2009 Jan; 67(1): 49–56.

Esmailzadeh A et al. Cholesterol-lowering effect of concentrated pomegranate juice consumption in type II diabetic patients with hyperlipidemia. *Int J Vitam Nutr Res* 2006 May; 76 (3): 147–51.

RED WINE

Brown et al. The biological responses to resveratrol and other polyphenols from alcoholic beverages. *Alcoholism Clin Exper Res* 2009.

Corder R. Red wine, chocolate and vascular health: developing the evidence base. *Heart* 2008 Jul; 94(7): 821–23.

Lu KT et al. Neuroprotective effects of resveratrol on cerebral ischemia-induced neuron loss mediated by free radical scavenging and cerebral blood flow elevation. *J Agric Food Chem* 2006 Apr 19; 54(8): 3126–31.

Olson ER et al. Inhibition of cardiac fibroblast proliferation and myofibroblast differentiation by resveratrol. *Am J Physiol Heart Circ Physiol* 2005 Mar; 288(3): H1131–38.

Renaud SC, et al. Moderate wine drinkers have lower hypertension-related mortality: a prospective cohort study in French men. *Am J Clin Nutr* 2004 Sep; 80(3): 621–25.

Waterhouse A. Saponins, a new cholesterol fighter, found in red wine. Study presented September 8, 2003, at the 226th national meeting of the American Chemical Society, September 7–11, 2003, NYC.

SALMON

Chrysohoou C et al. Long-term fish consumption is associated with protection against arrhythmia in healthy persons in a Mediterranean region—the ATTICA study. *Am J Clin Nutr* 2007 May; 85(5): 1385–91.

Connor W. Will the dietary intake of fish prevent atherosclerosis in diabetic women. *Am J Clin Nutr* 2004 Sep; 80(3): 626–32.

Erkkila A et al. Fish intake is associated with a reduced progression of coronary artery atherosclerosis in postmenopausal women with coronary artery disease. *Am J Clin Nutr*, 2004 Sep; 80(3): 626–32.

Holguin F et al. Cardiac autonomic changes associated with fish oil vs soy oil supplementation in the elderly. *Chest* 2005 Apr;127(4):1102–7.

Ueshima H et al. Food omega-3 fatty acid intake of individuals (total, linolenic acid, long-chain) and their blood pressure. INTERMAP Study. *Hypertension* 2007 Aug; 50(2): 313–39.

SWEET POTATOES

He, FJ, MacGregor GA. Beneficial effects of potassium on human health. *Physiol Plant* 2008 Aug; 133(4): 725–35.

Ye Z, Song H. Antioxidant vitamins intake and the risk of coronary heart disease: meta-analysis of cohort studies. *Eur J Cardiovasc Prev Rehabil* 2008 Feb; 15(1): 26–34.

TEMPEH

Jenkins DJ et al. Effect of plant sterols in combination with other cholesterol-lowering foods. *Metabolism* 2008 Jan; 57(1): 130–39.

Reynolds K et al. A meta-analysis of the effect of soy protein supplementation on serum lipids. *Am J Cardiol* 2006 Sept 1; 98(5): 633–40.

Taku K et al. Soy isoflavones lower serum total and LDL cholesterol in humans: a meta-analysis of 11 randomized controlled trials. *Am J Clin Nutr* 2007 Apr; 85(4): 1148–56.

TOFU

Reynolds K et al. A meta-analysis of the effect of soy proteins supplementation on serum lipids. *Am J Cardiol* 2006 Sep 1; 98(5): 633–40.

Taku K et al. Soy isoflavones lower serum total and LDL cholesterol in humans: a meta-analysis of 11 randomized controlled trials. *Am J Clin Nutr* 2007 Apr; 85(4): 1148–56.

TOMATOES

Lazarus SA, Bowen K, Garg ML. Tomato juice and platelet aggregation in type 2 diabetes. *JAMA* 2004 Aug 18; 292(7): 805–6.

Sesso HD, Liu S, Gaziano JM, Buring JE. Dietary lycopene, tomato-based food products and cardiovascular disease in women. *J Nutr* 2003 Jul; 133(7): 2336–41.

Silaste ML et al. Tomato juice decreases LDL cholesterol levels and increases LDL resistance to oxidation. *Br J Nutr* 2007 Dec; 98(6): 1251–58.

Visioli F et al. Protective activity of tomato products on in vivo markers of lipid oxidation. *Eur J Nutr* Aug; 42(4): 201–6.

Willcox JK et al. Tomatoes and cardiovascular health. *Crit Rev Food Sci Nutr* 2003; 43(1): 1–18.

TUNA

Boucher FR et al. Does selenium exert cardioprotective effects against oxidative stress in myocardial ischemia? *Acta Physiol Hung* 2008 Jun; 95(2): 187–94.

He K et al. Fish consumption and incidence of stroke: a meta-analysis of cohort studies. *Stroke* 2004 Jul; 35(7): 1538–42.

Holguin F et al. Cardiac autonomic changes associated with fish oil vs soy oil supplementation in the elderly. *Chest* 2005 Apr; 127(4): 1102–7.

Iso H et al. Intake of fish and omega-3 fatty acids and risk of stroke in women. *JAMA* 2001; 285(3): 304–12.

Mozaffarian D, et al. Fish intake and risk of incident atrial fibrillation. *Circulation* 2004 Jul 27; 110(4): 368–73.

WALNUTS

Anderson KJ et al. Walnut polyphenolics inhibit in vitro human plasma and LDL oxidation. *J Nutr* 131(11): 2837–42.

Fukuda T, Ito H, Yoshida T. Antioxidative polyphenols from walnuts (*Juglans regia L.*). *Phytochemistry*. 2003 Aug; 63(7): 795–801.

Kelly JH Jr, Sabate J. Nuts and coronary heart disease: an epidemiological perspective. *Br J Nutr* 2006 Nov; 96 Suppl 2: S61–67.

Marangoni F et al. Levels of the n-3 fatty acid eicosapentaenoic acid in addition to those of alpha linolenic acid are significantly raised in blood lipids by the intake of four walnuts a day in humans. *Nutr Metab Cardiovasc Dis* 2007 Jul; 17(6): 457–61.

Morgan JM et al. Effects of walnut consumption as part of a low-fat, low-cholesterol diet on serum cardiovascular risk factors. *Int J Vitam Nutr Res* 2002 Oct; 72(5): 341–47.

Zhao G et al. Dietary {alpha}-linolenic acid reduces inflammatory and lipid cardiovascular risk factors in hypercholesterolemic men and women. *J Nutr* 2004 Nov; 134(11): 2991–97.

WHEAT GERM

Calvo Romero, Lima Rodriguez EM. Natural treatments of hypercholesterolemia. *Rev Clin Esp* 2006 Nov; 206(10): 504–6.

Hargrove JL et al. Nutritional significance and metabolism of very long chain fatty alcohols and acids from dietary waxes. *Exp Biol Med* 2004 Mar; 229(3): 215–26.

Jenner A et al. Zinc supplementation inhibits lipid peroxidation and the development of atherosclerosis in rabbits fed a high cholesterol diet. *Free Radic Biol Med* 2007 Feb 15; 42(4): 559–66.

Leenhardt F et al. Wheat germ supplementation of a low vitamin E diet in rats affords effective antioxidant protection in tissues. *J Am Coll Nutr* 2008 Apr; 28(2): 222–28.

WINTER SQUASH

Riccioni G et al. Plasma antioxidants and asymptomatic carotid atherosclerotic disease. *Ann Nutr Metab* 2008; 53(2): 86–90.

Ylonen K et al. Dietary intakes and plasma concentrations of carotenoids and tocopherols in relation to glucose metabolism in subjects at high risk of type 2 diabetes: the Botnia Dietary Study. *Am J Clin Nutr* 2003 Jun; 76(6): 1434–41.

YOGURT

Engberink MF et al. Inverse association between dairy intake and hypertension: the Rotterdam Study. *Am J Clin Nutr* 2009 Jun; 89(6): 1877–83.

Fabian E, Elmadfa I. Influence of daily consumption of probiotic and conventional yoghurt on the plasma lipid profile in young healthy women. *Ann Nutr Metab* 2006; 50(4): 387–93.

Massey LK. Dairy food consumption, blood pressure and stroke. *J Nutr* 2001 Jul; 131(7): 1875–78.

Chapter 5
CARNITINE
Malaguarnera M et al. L-Carnitine supplementation reduces oxidized LDL cholesterol in patients with diabetes. *Am J Clin Nutr* 2009 Jan; 89(1): 71–76.

Schofield RS, Hill JA. Role of metabolically active drugs in the management of ischemic heart disease. *Am J Cardiovasc Drugs* 2001; 1(1): 23–35.

CAYENNE
Ahuja KD, Ball MJ. Effects of daily ingestion of chili on serum lipoprotein oxidation in adult men and women. *Br J Nutr* 2006 Aug; 96(2): 239–42.

Ahuja KD et al. The effect of 4-week chili supplementation on metabolic anc arterial function in humans. *Eur J Clin Nutr* 2007 Mar; 61(3): 326–33.

Sambaiah K, Satyanarayana MN. Hypocholesterolemic effect of red pepper & capsaicin. Indian J Exp Biol 1980 Aug;18(8): 898–99.

COENZYME Q10

Adarsh K et al. Coenzyme Q10 (CoQ10) in isolated dia-stolic heart failure in hypertrophic cardiomyopathy (HCM). *Biofactors* 2008; 32(1–4): 145–49.

Ankola DD et al. Development of potent oral nanoparticulate formulation of coenzyme Q10 for treatment of hypertension: can the simple nutritional supplements be used as first line therapeutic agents for prophylaxis/therapy? *Eur J Pharm Biopharm* 2007 Sep; 67(2): 361–69.

Judy WW et al. Myocardial preservation by therapy with coenzyme Q10 during heart surgery. *Clin Investig* 1993; 71(8 suppl): S155–61.

Keogh A et al. Randomised double-blind, placebo-controlled trial of coenzyme Q, therapy in class II and III systolic heart failure. *Heart Lung Circ* 2003; 12(3): 135–41.

Okello E et al. Combined statin/coenzyme Q10 as adjunctive treatment of chronic heart failure. *Med Hypotheses* 2009 Apr 29.

Pepe S et al. Coenzyme Q10 in cardiovascular disease. *Mitochondrion* 2007 Jun; 7 Suppl: S154–67.

D-RIBOSE

Illien S et al. Ribose improves myocardial function in congestive heart failure. *FASEB J* 2001; 15(5): A1142.

Muller C et al. Effect of ribose on cardiac adenine nucleotides in a donor model for heart transplantation. *Eur J Med Res* 1998 Dec 16; 3(12): 554–58.

Omran H et al. D-ribose improves diastolic function and quality of life in congestive heart failure patients: a prospective feasibility study. *Eur J Heart Failure* 2003; 5: 615–19.

Pliml W et al. Effects of ribose on exercise-induced ischaemia in stable coronary artery disease. *The Lancet* 1992; 340: 507–10.

GARLIC

Rahman K. Effects of garlic on platelet biochemistry and physiology. *Mol Nutr Food Res* 2007 Nov; 51(11): 1335–44.

Reinhart KM et al. The impact of garlic on lipid parameters: a systematic review and meta-analysis. *Nutr Res Rev* 2009 Jun; 22(1): 39–48.

Reinhart KM et al. Effects of garlic on blood pressure in patients with and without systolic hypertension: a meta-analysis. *Ann Pharmacother* 2008 Dec; 42(12): 1766–71.

GINGER

Nicoll R, Henein MY. Ginger (Zingiber officinale Roscoe): a hot remedy for cardiovascular disease? *Int J Cardiol* 2009 Jan 24; 131(3): 408–9.

Thomson M et al. The use of ginger (Zingiber officinale Rosc) as a potential anti-inflammatory and antithrombotic agent. *Prostaglandins Leukot Essent Fatty Acids* 2002 Dec; 67(6): 475–78.

Young HY et al. Synergistic effect of ginger and nifedipine on human platelet aggregation: a study in hypertensive patients and normal volunteers. *Am J Chin Med* 2006; 34(4): 545–51.

GINKGO BILOBA

Gardner CD et al. Effect of Ginkgo biloba (EGb 761) on treadmill walking time among adults with peripheral artery disease: a randomized clinical trial. *J Cardiopulm Rehabil Prev* 2008 Jul–Aug; 28(4): 258–65.

Wu YZ et al. Ginkgo biloba extract improves coronary artery circulation in patients with coronary artery disease: contribution of plasma nitric oxide and endothelin-1. *Phytother Res* 2008 Jun; 22(6): 734–39.

Wu Y et al. Ginkgo biloba extract improves coronary blood flow in healthy elderly adults: role of endothelium-dependent vasodilation. *Phytomedicine* 2008 Mar; 15(3): 164–69.

HAWTHORN

Holubarsch CJ et al. The efficacy and safety of Crataegus extract WS 1442 in patients with heart failure: the SPICE trial. *Eur J Heart Fail* 2008 Dec; 10(12): 1255–63.

Holubarsch CJ et al. Survival and prognosis: investigation of Crataegus extract WS 1442 in congestive heart failure (SPICE) rationale, study design and study protocol. *Eur J Heart Fail* 2000; 2(4): 431–37.

Leuchtgens H. Crataegus special extract WS1442 in heart failure, NYHA II. A placebo-controlled randomized double-blind study. *Fortschr Med* 1993; 111: 352–54.

Pittler MH et al. Hawthorn extract for treating chronic heart failure. *Cochrane Database Syst Rev* 2008 Jan 23; (1)CD005312.

Schmidt U et al. Efficacy of the hawthorn preparation LI132 in 78 patients with chronic congestive heart failure. *Phytomed* 1994; 1: 17–24.

Weikl A et al. Crataegus special extract WS 1442: objective proof of efficacy in patients with cardiac insufficiency (NYHA II). *Fortschr Med* 1996; 114: 291–96.

OMEGA-3 FATTY ACIDS

Holub BJ. Docosahexaenoic acid (DHA) and cardiovascular disease risk factors. *Prostaglandins Leukot Essent Fatty Acids* 2009 Jun 20.

Nestel P et al. The n-3 fatty acids eicosapentaenoic acid and docosahexaenoic acid increase systemic arterial compliance in humans. *Am J Clin Nutr* 2002; 76: 326–30.

Yokoyama M et al. Effects of eicosapentaenoic acid on major coronary events in hypercholesterolaemic patients (JELIS): a randomized, open-label, blinded endpoint analysis. *Lancet* 2007 Mar 31; 369(9567): 1090–98.

RED YEAST RICE

Becker DJ et al. Red yeast rice for dyslipidemia in statin-intolerance patients: a randomized trial. *Ann Intern Med* 2009 Jun 16; 150(12): 830–39.

Heber D et al. Cholesterol-lowering effects of a proprietary

Chinese red-yeast-rice dietary supplement. *Am J Clin Nutr* 1999; 69(2): 231–36.

Monograph. Monascus purpureus (red yeast rice). *Alt Med Rev* 2004; 9(2): 208–10.

Ong HT, Cheah JS. Statin alternatives or just placebo: an objective review of omega-3, red yeast rice and garlic in cardiovascular therapeutics. *Chin Med J (Engl)* 2008 Aug 20; 121(16): 1588–94.

RESVERATROL
Haider UG et al. Resveratrol increases serine 15-phosphorylated but transcriptionally impaired p53 and induces a reversible DNA replication block in serum-activated vascular smooth muscle cells. *Mol Pharmacol* 2003; 63(4): 925–32.

Olson ER et al. Inhibition of cardiac fibroblast proliferation and myofibroblast differentiation by resveratrol. *Am J Physiol Heart Circ Physiol* 2005 Mar; 288(3): H1131–38.

Wallerath T et al. Resveratrol, a olyphenolic phytoalexin present in red wine, enhances expression and activity of endothelial nitric oxide synthase. *Circulation* 2002 Sep 24; 106(13): 1652–58.

Wang SJ et al. Inhibitory effect of resveratrol on cardiac fibroblast proliferation induced by angiotensin II. *Zhongguo Zhong Xi Yi Jie He Za Zhi* 2008 Apr; 28(4): 334–38.

TURMERIC/CURCUMIN

Peschel D, et al. Curcumin induces changes in expression of genes involved in cholesterol homeostasis. *J Nutr Biochem* 2007 Feb; 18(2): 113–19.

Shah BH et al. Inhibitory effect of curcumin, a food spice from turmeric, on platelet-activating factor- and arachidonic acid-mediated platelet aggregation through inhibition of thromboxane formation and Ca2+ signaling. *Biochem Pharmacol* 1999 Oct 1; 58(7): 1167–72.

Soni KB, Kuttan R. Effect of oral curcumin administration on serum peroxides and cholesterol levels in human volunteers. *Indian J Physiol Pharmacol* 1992 Oct; 36(4): 273–75.

Srivastava G, Mehta JL. Currying the heart: curcumin and cardioprotection. *J Cardiovasc Pharmacol Ther* 2009 Mar; 14(1): 22–27.

Wongcharoen W, Phrommintikul A. The protective role of curcumin in cardiovascular diseases. *Int J Cardiol* 2009 Apr 3; 133(2): 145–51.

RESOURCES

American Heart Association
www.americanheart.org

American Heart Association Food Certification Program
checkmark.heart.org
Website that helps you create your own personal list of heart-healthy foods

American Society of Hypertension
www.ash-us.org
Professional and consumer level information on hypertension

Centers for Disease Control and Prevention
Website on heart disease
www.cdc.gov/heartdisease
Detailed information on heart disease and stroke, with many links

Consumer Reports
www.consumerreports.org/health/free-highlights/manage-your-health/choosing_supplements.htm
Article on "Five Steps to Choosing a Nutritional Supplement"

Kids Health—Heart Disease
kidshealth.org/kid/grownup/conditions/heart_disease.
html
A website that explains heart disease to children

Linus Pauling Institute
lpi.oregonstate.edu
Comprehensive information on vitamins, minerals, and
phytonutrients

Mayo Clinic
www.mayoclinic.com/health/heart-healthy-diet/nu00196
Mayo Clinic website that offers heart-healthy diet tips

National Heart, Lung, and Blood Institute
www.nhlbi.nih.gov/health/public/heart/chol/wyntk.htm
The NHLBI website with comprehensive information on
cholesterol

National Institutes of Health
Office of Dietary Supplements
ods.od.nih.gov/
Government-sponsored site that offers a wide variety of
information on dietary supplements and their use, safety,
latest news releases, and more

National Stroke Association
www.stroke.org
Lots of information on stroke prevention, recovery, and
risk factors

WomensHealth.gov
www.womenshealth.gov/FAQ/heart-healthy-eating.cfm
Government-sponsored website that provides heart-healthy information for women